Praise for *Agile Recipes*™ from *Re-Engineering the Kitchen*® Book Review

"One of the great additions to this book is that it doubles as a cookbook. Steele introduces the idea of Agile Recipes too, a term she coined to describe her streamlined recipes and cooking instructions. Unlike your favorite food blogs, this recipe doesn't come with a long intro about what this meal means to her and her family or any funny quips about how she's failed a million times to finally land on this perfect recipe.

It gives you only what you're looking for: the instructions, the ingredients, and the measurements. She throws in a picture or two for good measure but gets right to the meat of the task at hand: providing people with the simplest way to make food that aligns with their goals.

High nutritional content, low waste, and cost efficiency are at the top of Steele's priorities, and she nails them with over 100 Agile Recipes in this book."

– Independent Book Review October 2024

Full editorial review is available at independentbookreview.com

Cooking with Agile Recipes™

Real Food, Real Fast, Real Easy

Alin E. Steele, BSE, MBA, PE

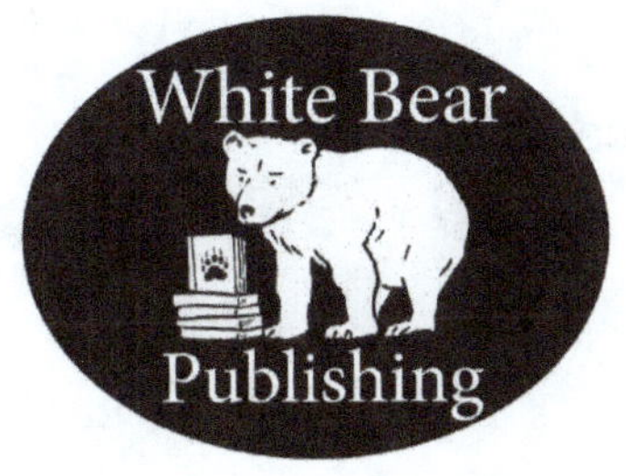

Cover Design: Simon Thompson

Interior Design: White Bear Publishing

Agile Character & Illustrations: Guy Harvey

Editor: White Bear Publishing

ISBN-13: 979-8-9893475-5-1

Library of Congress Control Number: 2025917515

First Edition – September 2025
Printed in the United States of America

Published by White Bear Publishing
Ramsey, MN

Table of Contents

INTRODUCTION

What if we could make cooking a little easier? What if it was a little quicker? Involved less wasted food? How about less clean up? Would you be willing to cook a little more often?

How about if it was easier to cook more real food with less ultra-processed ingredients? What if I told you that you could save time and money by making more things from scratch? Would you be interested in learning more?

There are many recipes that boast being "quick and easy." Maybe they have limited ingredients and simple steps. That's a good start but maybe we can do better.

Let's start with a blank sheet of paper and re-engineer the basic recipe format to be much more functional and suited to the 21st century. What if we created a new standard recipe format that was intuitive and gave you all the information on one sheet or one screen? Imagine being able to figure out if a recipe was going to work for you at a glance! No more wasted time hunting for the actual recipe and then reading three pages of unnecessarily detailed instructions.

What if we made the recipes flexible by showing you possible ingredient substitutions right up front? How about giving you options to vary the basic recipe to achieve different results? One recipe could give you the same info that would take who-knows-how-long comparing several recipes on the internet.

Now that we have a new recipe format, what if we developed recipes to minimize the number of ingredients and streamline the number of steps? Wouldn't this save time all around? What if we sized the recipes to match standard food packaging? Wouldn't this result in less food waste? How about if we designed steps to minimize the equipment needed? Every item we avoid using saves time and effort; from getting it out, using it, washing it, and then putting it back away.

Lastly, what if we made it easier to find recipe ideas for the whole food ingredients we have on hand? What if there were easy charts where we could look up, say, a certain veggie and see that there are several recipes to choose from?

The answers to all of these "What if" questions are right here in this book. Agile Recipes™ have been designed to make cooking Real Food more efficient in every sense. Let's make it easier to spend less time, money, and effort on better food!

Some thoughts on nutrition . . .

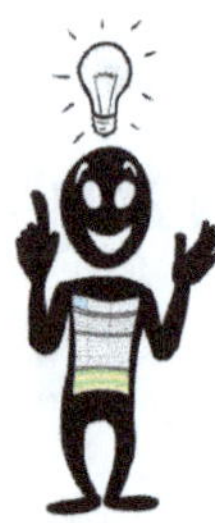

"Let food be your medicine and medicine be your food."
– Hippocrates

"I don't think I'll ever grow old and say, 'What was I thinking eating all those fruits and vegetables?" – Nancy S. Mure

"I believe in eating real food." – Martha Stewart

"Those who think they have no time for healthy eating will sooner or later have to find time for illness." – Edward Stanley

"Don't eat anything your great-grandmother wouldn't recognize as food."
– Michael Pollan

"To eat is a necessity, but to eat intelligently is an art."
– La Rochefoucauld

CHAPTER 1

WHY AGILE RECIPES™?

Agile Recipes™ were developed to make it easier to cook more Real Food at home. Whether following a vegan, vegetarian, carnivore, low carb, low fat, or just an average diet style, many people strive to eat more whole foods and less ultra-processed junk. It is a worthwhile goal but who has the time or energy to cook that much? It feels like a major project just to figure out what to cook, with the ingredients, time, and resources on hand. Then, once you have decided what to prepare, you still need to get it on the table and then clean up afterward.

In my book ***Re-Engineering the Kitchen®: A Simple Method to put Real Food you your table faster, easier and cheaper***, I present a straightforward process to develop a food plan based on individual goals including nutritional basics, shopping guidelines, easy preparation, and efficient kitchen management. The Agile Recipes™ contained here were developed to support the ***Re-Engineering the Kitchen®*** goals of making healthier food easier to achieve.

Nutrition

By now we have all gotten the message that ultra-processed foods (UPF) are linked to, if not the cause of, many of the non-communicable diseases that plague our western society (obesity, metabolic disease, CHD, etc.). It is estimated that Americans get an alarming 60-70% of their calories from ultra-processed foods. UPFs are hard to avoid but reducing UPF intake is a high priority for many people. The Agile Recipes™ here give you easy options to make Real Food at home rather than buying a commercially prepared UPF. It is easier than you have been led to believe, and you will save money in the process.

It is important to understand what ultra-processed food is. The NOVA classification was developed by the researchers at the University of Sao Paulo to define the extent of processing of foods. Figure 1 on the following page summarizes the four NOVA classifications.

Figure 1 – The NOVA Food Classification System

Group	Classification	Food Groups
1	Unprocessed or minimally processed foods	Fruit, vegetables, legumes, milk, eggs, yogurt, meat, nuts, poultry, seafood, grains and flours, spices, tea, juice, coffee, and water.
2	Processed culinary ingredients	Salt, white and brown sugar, honey, vegetable oils, butter, lard, and coconut fat.
3	Processed foods	Condensed milk, cream, cheese, traditionally cured ham and bacon, canned fruit, canned vegetables, canned fish, freshly made unpackaged bread, beer, cider, and wine.
4	Ultra-Processed Foods	Processed meats, ice cream, breakfast cereals, pizza, margarine, commercially baked breads and pastries, cookies, chips, chocolate, candies, carbonated drinks, instant soups, milkshakes, mayonnaise, fruit drinks, artificially sweetened drinks, and pudding/custard.

Reference: *Monteiro CA, Cannon G, Moubarac JC, Levy RB, Louzada MLC, Jaime PC. The UN Decade of Nutrition, the NOVA food classification and the trouble with ultra-processing. Public Health Nutr. 2018 Jan;21(1):5-17. doi: 10.1017/S1368980017000234. Epub 2017 Mar 21. PMID: 28322183; PMCID: PMC10261019. pubmed.ncbi.nlm.nih.gov/28322183/.*

If you ever wonder whether a certain food is just "processed" or is it "ultra-processed," read the label and ask yourself "Could I make this in my home kitchen?" If the answer is "No," then it is probably an UPF.

Agile Recipes™ have been developed with a focus on whole foods and minimal use of highly processed ingredients like mixes, packaged foods, and industrial seed oils. They include homemade versions of many items that are often ultra-processed including baked goods, desserts, salad dressings, sauces, and marinades.

Efficiency

The entire point of Agile Recipes™ is to make it easier to prepare delicious Real Food.

The easier it is to cook, the more likely it is to happen.

To improve efficiency, we have squeezed out little bits of time, money, and effort at each step in the process.

Improvements with Agile Recipes™

1. Quick and easy to decide what to prepare
   a. Simple charts to find preparation options for your ingredients
   b. Scope of recipes are intuitive at a glance
   c. Substitutions are listed in the recipe
2. Streamlined Recipes
   a. A one-page, intuitive layout
   b. Minimal steps
   c. Minimal ingredients
   d. Minimal equipment
   e. Flex information included
   f. Minimized processed ingredients
3. Reduced cost and waste
   a. Basic ingredients not expensive limited-use ingredients
   b. Substitutions and variations - use what you have
   c. Recipes tailored to package size
   d. Reduce waste by making the amount you'll use

Go ahead and commit to buying and cooking more of those healthy foods: Agile Recipes™ have you covered!

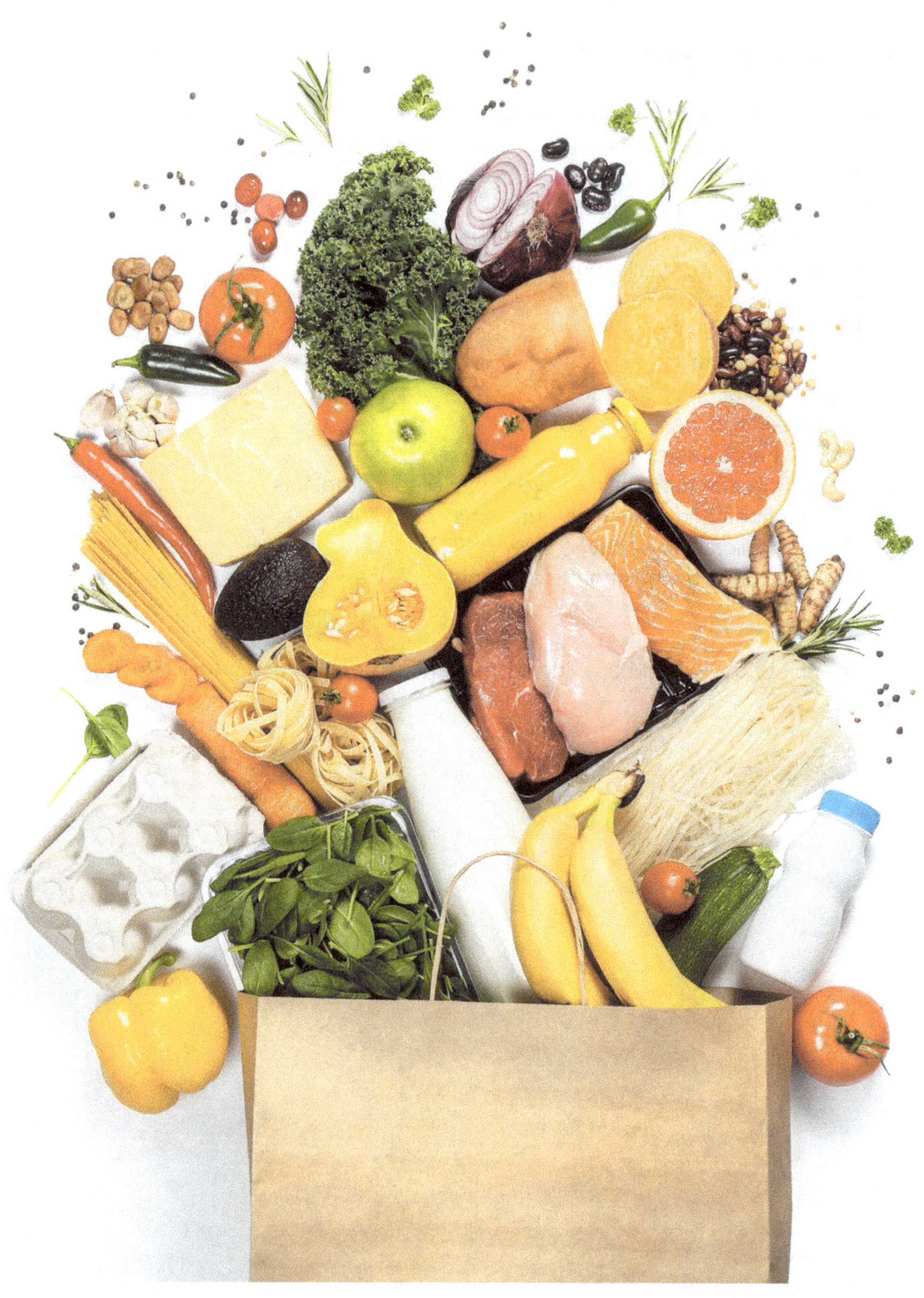

CHAPTER 2

What to Cook?

A recent meme floating around social media bemoans the aspect of "adulting" that now one must figure out what to cook – every single day for the rest of your life. It can feel a bit overwhelming.

Let's presume that you have ingredients on hand and are looking for preparation ideas. If you are going to put the effort into cooking food at home, you'd probably like it to be delicious and as healthy as possible. If you are like most people, you have a limited amount of time and energy to spend on this daily effort.

Included in this book are recipes that focus on simple ways to prepare many of the most common whole foods, including protein and produce. To make the process quick and easy, we have developed "What to do with ____" charts. These charts allow you to look up recipe options by key ingredients. For example, if you look up broccoli, you'll find four recipes to choose from. These charts also allow you to cross-reference the recipes to see potential variations in the key ingredients. For example, the recipe for Enchilada Surprise shows that it can be made with a variety of different proteins. This means that you can always purchase the best ingredients, confident that you have quick and easy preparation ideas handy.

Use the following "What to Do with ___" charts to quickly find recipe ideas for your ingredients.

- Figure 2 - What to do with Meat
- Figure 3 - What to do with Legumes, Eggs, and Dairy
- Figure 4 - What to do with Fruit and Grains
- Figure 5 - What to do with Vegetables

Page #	Figure 2 What to do With Meat	Ground Beef	Steak	Skirt or Flank Steak	Canned Chicken	Ground Chicken	Chicken Breast Bnls	Chicken on Bone	Turkey (include ground)	Pork (include sausage)	Leftover/Cooked Meat	Shrimp and Crab	Canned Tuna	Fresh Fish
82	5-Minute Flatbread^{V} – 4 Ways						X			X	X			
83	Apricot Glazed Pork Tenderloin									X				
84	Asian Glazed Anything^{V}		X				X			X	X	X		
85	Baked Rice Casserole^{V}				X	X	X	X	X	X	X			
86	Balsamic Glazed Chicken						X							
154	Beans and Rice^{V}									X				
87	Beef Stroganoff	X	X											
49	Biscuits and Gravy									X				
50	Breakfast Sausage					X			X	X				
36	Buffalo Chicken Dip				X		X	X			X			
89	Chicken Curry – 2 Ways				X		X	X	X		X			
90	Chicken Divan				X	X	X		X					
91	Chicken Mushroom Marsala						X				X			
92	Chicken Paillard						X							
93	Chicken Paprika						X	X						
94	Chicken Salad – 4 Ways						X	X						
95	Chili Express	X	X			X			X		X			
96	Citrus Grilled Shrimp											X		
97	Crab Cakes											X		
99	Enchilada Surprise^{V} – 3 Ways	X			X	X	X	X	X	X	X			
100	Fajitas		X	X			X	X				X		
101	Fried Rice^{V}						X			X	X			
102	Hammered Chops									X				

Page #	**Figure 2** **What to do With Meat**	Ground Beef	Steak	Skirt or Flank Steak	Canned Chicken	Ground Chicken	Chicken Breast Bnls	Chicken on Bone	Turkey (include ground)	Pork (include sausage)	Leftover/Cooked Meat	Shrimp and Crab	Canned Tuna	Fresh Fish
103	Italian Sausage – Scratch					X			X	X				
105	Lemon Butter Baked Fish													X
107	Marinated Flank Steak			X										
108	Meatballs – Italian	X				X			X	X				
109	Meatloaf – 5 Ways	X				X			X	X				
110	Oven-Fried Chicken – 4 Ways						X							
136	Pasta Salad[V] – 4 Ways												X	
113	Picadillo	X								X				
114	Poached Chicken						X	X				X		X
115	Roast Pork Tenderloin									X				
116	Salmon - Glazed 3 Ways													
57	Sausage Brunch Bake								X	X				
117	Shrimp and Cheesy Grits											X		
118	Shrimp Scampi											X		
119	Sloppy Joes	X				X			X					
120	Spaghetti Sauce w/ Meat	X				X			X	X				
122	Tacos	X	X			X	X		X	X	X			
123	Teriyaki for All		X	X			X			X		X		
124	Tuna Cake												X	
138	Tuna Salad Niçoise												X	
125	Tuna Salad – 2 Ways												X	
126	Yogurt Marinated Chicken						X	X						

Page #	Figure 3 What to do With Legumes, Eggs, and Dairy	Chickpeas	Black Beans	Lentils	Red Beans	White Beans	Eggs	Cheese	Cottage Cheese/Ricotta	Milk/Cream	Tofu
152	**$100 Macaroni & Cheese[V]**							X	X	X	
82	**5-Minute Flatbread[V] – 4 Ways**							X			
84	**Asian Glazed Aything[V]**										X
85	**Baked Rice Casserole – 3 Ways**						X	X		X	
35	**Baked Salsa Dip[V]**							X			
130	**Bean Salad[V] – 4 Ways**	X	X		X	X					
183	**Bean Soup Express**		X		X	X					
154	**Beans and Rice[V] – 3 Ways**		X		X						
88	**Black Bean & Sweet Potato Chili[V]**		X								
64	**Bread Pudding[V] – 5 Ways**						X			X	
37	**Cheese Fondue[V]**							X		X	
95	**Chili Express**		X		X	X					
159	**Continental Beans[V]**		X		X	X					
38	**Crispy Chickpea Snacks[V] – 4 Ways**	X									
51	**Egg Cups[V] – 5 Ways**						X	X	X		
69	**Egg Custard[V]**						X			X	
53	**French Toast Casserole[V]**						X		X	X	

Page #	Figure 3 What to do With Legumes, Eggs, and Dairy	Chickpeas	Black Beans	Lentils	Red Beans	White Beans	Eggs	Cheese	Cottage Cheese/Ricotta	Milk/Cream	Tofu
101	Fried Rice[V]						X				X
35	Hummus[V]	X									
104	Lasagna Florentine[V]						X	X	X		
106	Lentils del Sol[V]			X							
186	Lentil Soup[V] – 5 Ways			X							
74	Milk Pudding[V] – 5 Ways						X			X	
112	Palak Paneer[V]							X			
55	Potato Frittata[V] – 4 Ways						X	X			
174	Rice Pilaf[V] – 4 Ways							X			
77	Rice Pudding[V] – 2 Ways						X			X	
56	Ricotta Pancakes[V]						X		X		
78	Ricotta Cheesecake[V]						X		X		
57	Sausage Brunch Bake						X	X		X	
178	Savory White Beans[V]					X					
58	Spinach Mushroom Bake[V]						X	X	X		
121	Stuffed Shells[V]						X	X	X		
59	Swedish Pancakes[V]						X			X	

Page #	Figure 4 What to do With Fruit and Grain	Apple	Applesauce	Banana	Dried Fruit	Fresh Berries	Frozen Berries	Peach, Plum, Apricot	Pineapple	Bread, Tortillas	Oats	Rice, Quinoa	Flour, Wheat, Pasta, etc.
152	$100 Macaroni & Cheese^{V}												X
82	5-Minute Flatbread^{V} – 4 Ways									X			
60	Applesauce Oatmeal Crisp^{V}		X		X						X		
85	Baked Rice Casserole^{V}											X	
42	Banana Bread^{V}			X									X
61	Bananas Foster^{V}			X									
62	Banana Pudding Parfait^{V}			X									
154	Beans and Rice^{V} – 3 Ways											X	
43	Beer Bread^{V}												X
44	Biscuits/Shortcake^{V} – 5 Ways												X
63	Brandied Peaches^{V}							X					
64	Bread Pudding^{V} – 5 Ways				X					X			
66	Brownies^{V}												X
67	Butter Berry Cobbler^{V}					X	X	X					X
132	Carrot Salad w/ Fruit^{V}	X			X				X				
68	Chocolate Applesauce Cake^{V}		X		X								X
45	Corn Bread^{V}												X
70	Essential Cake^{V} – 6 Ways												X
71	Fast Fruit Filling^{V}					X	X	X					

Page #	Figure 4 What to do With Fruit and Grain	Apple	Applesauce	Banana	Dried Fruit	Fresh Berries	Frozen Berries	Peach, Plum, Apricot	Pineapple	Bread, Tortillas	Oats	Rice, Quinoa	Flour, Wheat, Pasta, etc.
101	Fried Rice[V]											X	
53	French Toast Casserole[V]						X			X			
46	Irish Soda Bread[V]												X
47	No Touch Bread[V]												X
54	Oatmeal Pancakes[V]										X		X
136	Pasta Salad [V] – 4 Ways												X
75	Pantry Cake[V]												X
171	Pineapple Casserole[V]								X				
76	Pumpkin Muffins[V]												X
174	Rice Pilaf [V] – 4 Ways											X	
77	Rice Pudding[V] – 2 Ways				X							X	
137	Rice Salad[V] – 3 Ways											X	
56	Ricotta Pancakes[V]												X
79	Russian Tea Cakes[V]												X
80	Spiced Poached Fruit[V]	X						X	X				
59	Swedish Pancakes[V]												X
122	Tacos, Tostadas, Enchiladas									X			
48	Yeast Rolls[V]												X

Page #	Figure 5 What to do With Vegetables	Avocado	Baby Bok Choy	Broccoli	Brussels Sprouts	Collard Greens	Kale	Salad Greens	Spinach
82	5-Minute Flatbread[V]								X
153	Aloo Gobi[V]								
130	Bean Salad[V] – 4 Ways								
183	Bean Soup Express[V]								
88	Black Bean and Sweet Potato Chili[V]								
155	Braised Cabbage[V]								
131	Brussels Sprouts Salad[V]				X				
132	Carrot Salad w/ Fruit[V]								
156	Cauliflower & Sweet Potato Curry[V]								
157	Cauliflower Marinara[V]								
158	Citrus Glazed Brussels Sprouts[V]				X				
144	Classic Marinara Sauce[V]								
184	Cream of Mushroom Soup[V]								
160	Creamed Vegetables[V]								X
133	Cucumber Salads[V]								
146	Enchilada Sauce[V]								
99	Enchilada Surprise[V]								
185	French Onion Soup[V]								
101	Fried Rice[V]								
161	Frizled Cabbage[V] – 3 Ways								
162	Glazed Carrots[V] – 4 Ways								
134	Green Bean Salad w/ Goat Cheese[V]								
163	Green Beans[V] – 4 Ways								
164	Green Bean Sucotash[V]								

Cabbage	Cauliflower	Cucumber	Green Beans	Mushrooms	Onions	Summer Squash	Bell Peppers	Carrots	Spaghetti Squash	Sweet Potato	Winter Squash	Corn	Peas	Potato	Tomatoes
				X	X		X								X
	X													X	
			X												
					X			X						X	
					X					X					X
X					X			X							
								X							
	X														
	X									X					X
					X										X
				X											
X	X		X	X								X	X	X	
		X													
					X										X
										X		X			
					X										
					X			X					X		
X					X			X							
								X							
			X												
			X	X											
			X									X			

Page #	Figure 5 What to do With Vegetables	Avocado	Baby Bok Choy	Broccoli	Brussels Sprouts	Collard Greens	Kale	Salad Greens	Spinach
165	Green Bean Un-Casserole[V]								
39	Guacamole Fresca[V]	X							
166	Lemon Bacon Brussels Sprouts[V]				X				
167	Lemon Garlic Kale[V]						X		
168	Mediterranean Spaghetti Squash[V]								
170	Moroccan Cauliflower[V]								
135	Napa Cabbage Salad[V]								
188	Potato Broccoli Soup[V]			X					
55	Potato Frittata[V]								X
172	Quick Creamed Spinach[V]								X
173	Quick Spaghetti Squash[V]								
174	Rice Pilaf[V] - 4 Ways			X					
175	Roasted Vegetables[V] – 5 Ways			X	X				
177	Sautéed Baby Bok Choy[V]		X						
179	Simple Greens[V]					X			
180	Spinach – Flash Sautéed[V]								X
58	Spinach Mushroom Bake[V]								X
40	Spinach Bites[V]								X
181	Sweet Potato Casserole[V]								
138	Tuna Salad Niçoise							X	
182	Vegetables au Gratin[V]			X					
189	Vegetable Soup[V]						X		

Cabbage	Cauliflower	Cucumber	Green Beans	Mushrooms	Onions	Summer Squash	Bell Peppers	Carrots	Spaghetti Squash	Sweet Potato	Winter Squash	Corn	Peas	Potato	Tomatoes
			X												
					X										X
					X	X	X		X						X
	X														
X															
														X	
														X	
					X										
					X				X						
				X	X			X					X		
	X			X	X	X	X	X		X	X			X	
				X											
										X					
			X											X	X
	X							X		X				X	
X			X		X			X				X	X	X	X

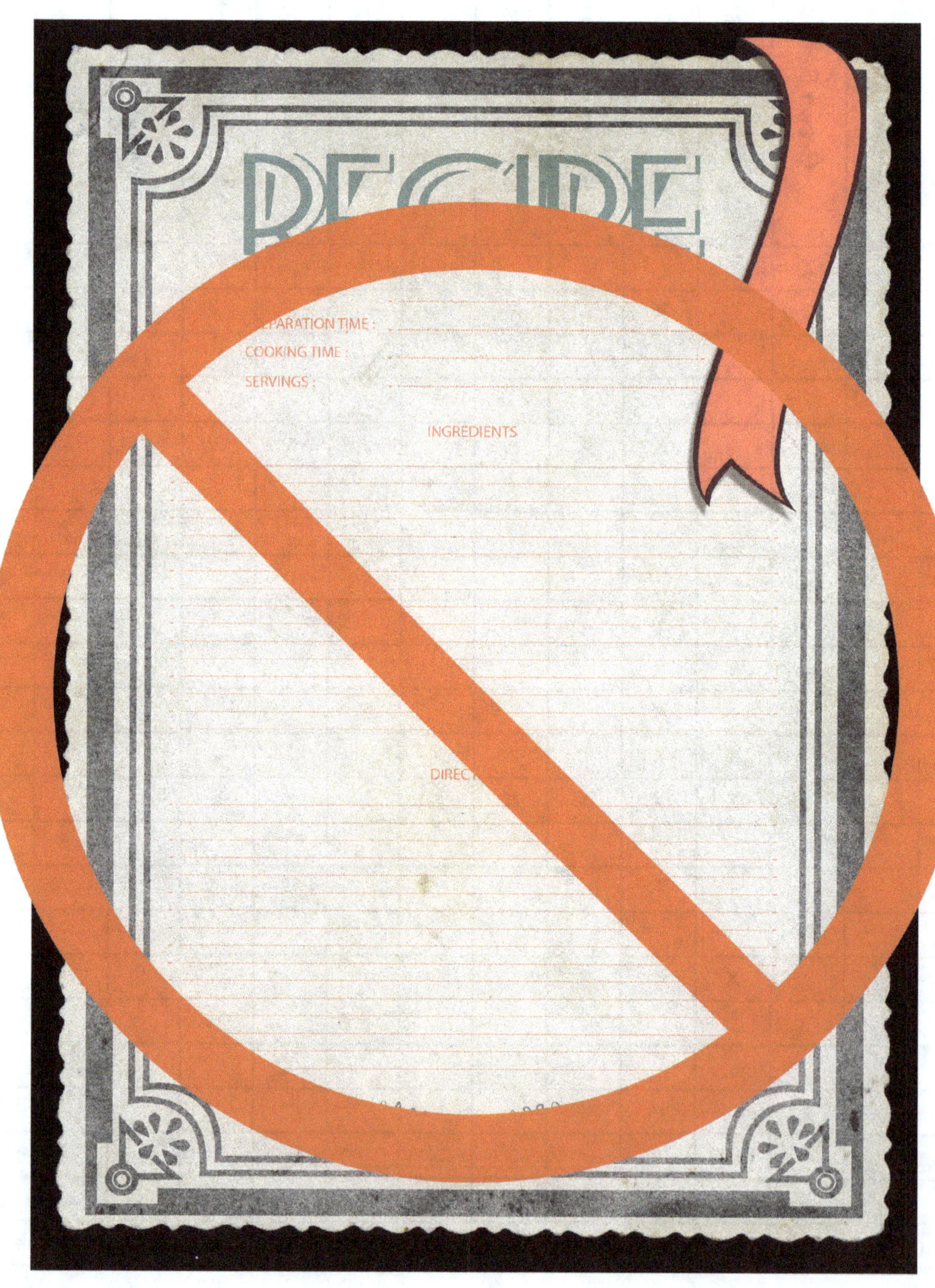
RECIPE
COOKING TIME :
SERVINGS :
INGREDIENTS

CHAPTER 3

INTRODUCING AGILE RECIPES™

In my book ***Re-Engineering the Kitchen®: A simple method to put Real Food on your table faster, easier, and cheaper***, I introduced the concept of an entirely new recipe design. Agile Recipes™ were created to make it quicker and easier for the cook to find a workable recipe and prepare more Real Food from the ingredients they have on hand. The recipes in this book are focused on simple ways to prepare healthy dishes and homemade alternatives to ultra-processed foods. However, these recipes are not just "easy", they have been completely redesigned to be efficient and flexible. These recipes are a tool to help you prepare Real Food more often.

The Best Recipe

How is it that, with the proliferation of recipes from cookbooks, online recipe collections, magazines, and television shows, we still struggle to find the right recipe? I get food magazines and have a healthy collection of cookbooks, recipe cards, and stacks of loose paper recipes, complete with hand-scribbled notes and petrified food stains. I enjoy just reading recipes and I often learn some new techniques or flavor combinations. That doesn't mean I will ever make any of these recipes. Frequently, the recipe just doesn't fit my situation. It is too long and complicated. It has an ingredient that I am unlikely to buy, and I am unsure if the recipe will tolerate a substitution. I can't envision a scenario where I would purchase $25 worth of fresh herbs for a single dish. Or maybe something doesn't look "right" – so I waste time looking at other recipes for the same thing, trying to judge if the proportions are correct. Or worse, I go down the Internet rabbit hole of reading recipe reviews. Before I realize it, I have spent an improbable amount of time trying to find a recipe that works for the pork chops I need to cook right now.

I have many beloved recipes that are long and intricate; they require precise proportions and exact procedures. If I am going to make those dishes, I need to take the time to make them right. They may not happen often but, when they do, they play to rave reviews. Crème Brûlée, Cassoulet and my mothers-in-law's scratch spaghetti sauce for example. These may be wonderful recipes, but you will not find them here in this book. They are too complicated, time-consuming, and inflexible.

How do you judge a recipe? It goes without saying that the result must be delicious. Other than that, the best recipe is the one that suits the situation at hand.

Updated Recipe Format

The format of recipes has changed very little in centuries. You can easily understand historical cookbooks, an attribute that makes them charming souvenirs. We may find the outdated terminology quaint (a thumb of butter, or glass of sugar), but the basic format is familiar to us: a list of ingredients then instructions. While this format has enjoyed centuries of acceptance and success, it does leave room for improvement. We have improved many of our processes at home, school, and work and, along with that, we have improved our communication and documentation of those processes. Think of all the instructions that have become visually accessible and intuitive: clothing and food labels, web navigation, electronic device operations, and DIY furniture assembly to name just a few.

Features to improve the old recipe format would include:

- Make it easy to understand the scope of the recipe at a glance.
- Clearly show the essential ingredients and possible substitutions.
- List options separate from the basic recipe.
- Ensure it is visually accessible – your eyes quickly find the information you seek.
- Keep it brief – eliminate unnecessary information.
- Be consistent with layout so the same information is always in the same place.

These format changes will improve the recipe by communicating more information and doing so more efficiently.

Streamlined Process

Whenever I cook, I am always looking for process-improvement opportunities. At each step, I am considering what value that action or ingredient adds. Can I consolidate steps? Is it really necessary to list oil as an ingredient when it is just a pan lubrication? Do you really need to mix the dry ingredients in a separate bowl? Can you make this without the special-purpose equipment? How can clean-up be minimized? How can we minimize wasted ingredients? (I hate it when a recipe calls for a partial container of something!) Which ingredients can be omitted or substituted?

All the recipes in this book are designed to taste great yet be simple, reliable, flexible, and forgiving. They have been re-engineered to achieve our many objectives, including reducing waste.

Process improvement changes have been made to:

- Minimize steps and effort.
- Use commonly available ingredients and list substitutions.
- Include information to meet some dietary requirements.
- Proportion recipe to fit common package sizes.
- Reduce the required equipment to the minimum and include low-tech options.
- Minimize the amount of kitchen clean-up required.

Why streamline a recipe at all?

Most recipes have been developed utilizing standard techniques to achieve an optimal end result with no regard to the time and resource constraints of the average person trying to feed their family. The most delicious recipe in the world is of no use if you don't have the time to make it. Traditional biscuit recipes, for example, require many steps using a pastry cutter, multiple bowls and measuring cups, a pastry board and rolling pin, etc., resulting in a second "project" to clean-up afterward! The streamlined recipe for biscuits used here only requires a single glass bowl (or large measuring cup), a knife, a measuring cup and spoon, and a scoop as shown in the photo below: low impact and minimal clean-up.

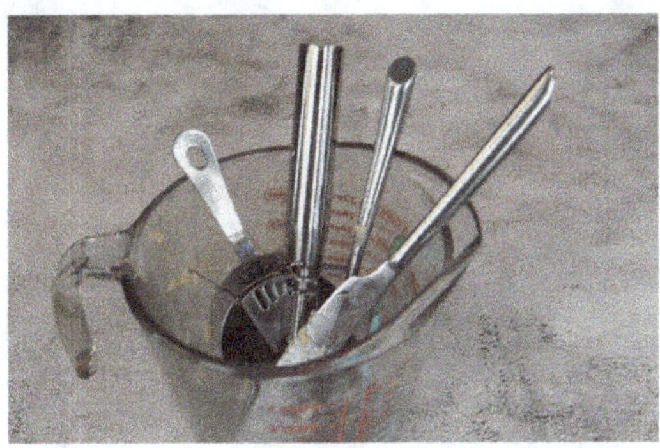

Guide to Agile Recipes™

Every Agile Recipe™ follows the same, intuitive layout so that information is accessible at a glance. The graphic features make it easier to find the information as you look back and forth between your cooking and the Agile Recipe™. The one-page layout will display concisely on paper or the screen of your device (download PDFs of Agile Recipes™ at www.ReEngineeringtheKitchen.com). A sample recipe is shown on the following page.

Figure 6 – Sample Agile Recipe™

New Graphic Layout
Visually Accessible at a Glance
Intuitive and Consistent

Key Ingredient Type — **Substitutions** — **Type of Dish**

GRAIN	**Biscuit/Shortcake**[V] **Makes 6 Biscuits**	**BREAD**
INGREDIENTS		**SUBSTITUTE**
3 Tbsp	Butter	Crisco or margarine
1½ C	Flour (180 g)	1 C rice flour + ½ C tapioca flour (GF) or substitute up to 50% whole grain flour
½ Tbsp	Baking powder	
½ Tbsp	Sugar	Brown sugar or dry sugar substitute
½ tsp	Salt	
½ C	Milk	Half & Half or buttermilk or half cream/half water
STEPS		
1	Preheat oven to 400°F. Grease pan or line with parchment.	
2	In a heat-proof glass bowl or 4 C glass measuring cup, warm butter to room temp in micro.	
3	Add flour to bowl with butter. If you have a scale, weigh flour directly into your bowl.	
4	Add baking powder, salt and sugar to flour. Stir to distribute dry ingredients.	
5	With a fork, work the flour mixture and butter together until it becomes coarse and grainy.	
6	Add milk and stir just enough to fully incorporate.	
7	Use scoop or spoon to make 6 rounded biscuits. Each should be about 1½ inches high.	
8	Bake for 12-18 minutes, until golden brown at edges.	
9	Store covered. May reheat for 5 minutes in 350° F oven or 15 seconds in micro.	
OPTIONS		
A	**Rolled Biscuits:** Roll dough on floured surface to about ¾ inch thickness. Cut with cookie cutter or with a glass or jar of desired diameter.	
B	**Cheese Biscuits:** Stir in ½ C any shredded cheese into dough. Can add ½ tsp garlic powder to dry ingredients for more savory flavor.	
C	**Cinnamon Bun Biscuits:** Place biscuits close together in 9" pan, flatten each slightly by hand. Mix 2 Tbsp soft butter with 1 tsp cinnamon and 2 Tbsp sugar. Spread paste over biscuits prior to baking.	
D	**Shortcake:** Add another ½ Tbsp of sugar to the dough. For decoration, brush with butter and sprinkle with sugar prior to baking.	

Essential Ingredients (INGREDIENTS) — **Streamlined Steps** (STEPS) — **Variations** (OPTIONS)

Agile Recipes™ will give the basic recipe and then several variations or options, so you can make it work for you. The variations might suggest additional ingredients, variable flavor combinations, options using store-bought vs. homemade components, sweet and savory renditions, or a list of compatible ingredients.

Referring to the sample Biscuit/Shortcake Agile Recipe™ on the previous page, here are some of the features that make it an Agile Recipe™ compared to a typical recipe:

Revised Process:

- Use only one prep bowl:
  Use tempered glass so cold or frozen butter can be microwaved.
  Measure dry ingredients directly into the bowl with butter. Incorporate baking powder and salt by stirring into flour while on top of the butter.
- Use scale to measure flour – increases accuracy, less measuring overspill, and no measuring cup to wash.
- Use a fork to cut in flour and butter (eliminates hard-to-clean pastry cutter).
- Use a scoop or rounded spoon to get rounded biscuits – eliminates messy rolling but looks better than "drop biscuits".

Substitutions:

» Substitutions for different fats.
» Proportions for common gluten-free flour.
» Substitutions for milk.

Options:

- Option to make a sweeter shortcake.
- Can be rolled and cut for a fancier presentation.
- Savory cheese biscuits.
- Cinnamon bun biscuits.

Would I use this recipe when hosting a fancy brunch? Absolutely. Perhaps I would "flex" it toward the higher-end result by using buttermilk and rolling/cutting the biscuits for a prettier presentation. On the other hand, I am willing to make the basic version of these biscuits at the drop of a hat because they can be so easy and low impact. I have never had anyone turn down a fresh biscuit, hot out of the oven. The "best" recipe is the one that meets your needs at the moment.

Why is this collection of Agile Recipes™ unique?

What is the difference between this collection of recipes and other cookbooks, websites, and cooking shows? The Agile Recipes™ here are included for one reason and one reason only: to help you put Real Food on your table faster, easier, and cheaper. This means having easy preparation methods for healthy dishes and homemade options for often ultra-processed foods. There is no discussion of the recipe's origin or history. There is no charming story about Aunt Bertie making this dish for every holiday. There is no lengthy description of technique or pictures of the steps. I admit that I do enjoy reading such things elsewhere, but not when I need to get a meal prepared right now. The two approaches to presenting recipes represent two entirely different objectives.

This makes sense when you consider that we are now living in the "Attention Economy", a term coined by political scientist Herbert A. Simon. Our most valuable companies are those that command your attention the most effectively. Everyone who develops and delivers content is trying to make money from ads. Most food-related content is developed primarily as entertainment, with a modicum of information for value. They make money by maintaining your attention. This applies to everyone from the busy-mom-with-a-cooking-website to the multi-channel behemoths with a print, web, and television presence. With this perspective in mind, you can see that efficiency is not aligned with the objective of maintaining attention for the longest time. It is not to say that one approach is inherently better or worse – it just means that they are different.

Another way that this collection of Agile Recipes™ is different than the norm is how the recipes are structured. Agile Recipes™ have a "Theme and Variation" structure. Historically, each normal recipe leads to a singular outcome. For instance, making tacos with ground chicken, turkey, or beef would involve at least three distinct recipes (or more if you can find ways to vary the recipe and photos with different accents). The Agile Recipe™ for Tacos is one "theme" recipe, with several "variations" outlined. It is a waste of the readers' time to repeat the same core information multiple times – and make them hunt and peck to find what they need. But remember, commandeering your time is their primary objective! How many ads did you view while you were sifting through six recipes?

You can always quickly find the Agile Recipe™ you want because they are categorized several different ways:

- By key ingredient in the "What to do with ______" charts on pages 8-17
- Listed by the type of dish on pages 29-34
- Index in the back of the book

The unique Theme and Variation structure of Agile Recipes™ requires a new way of organizing the recipes. First, we organize the recipes around the primary ingredients: Vegetables, Protein (meat), Protein (other), Fruits and Grains. Protein (meat) includes beef, pork, poultry, and fish. Protein (other) includes dairy products, eggs, and legumes. You may notice that many recipes have ingredients from multiple categories, but we choose the primary to be the most prevalent ingredients. Use the "What to do with ____" charts in Chapter 2 to look up all the recipes that work for your key ingredient. This allows us to efficiently find preparation alternatives for the foods you have on hand. Next, the recipes are categorized by the type of dish, e.g. Main, Side, Dessert, etc.

Also included are recipes for Marinades & Brines, Salad Dressings, and Sauces. There are Agile Recipes™ for several key "from scratch" sauces. However, the rest of the recipes for each category are so super-simple and quick to assemble that they are presented in charts. There are charts for:

- Marinades & Brines
- Salad Dressings
- Sauces

This makes it very easy to review and then quickly prepare one. The charts list the ingredients and instructions as needed.

Notes about Agile Recipes™

The recipes included here start with very basic ingredients and are average American in their taste. While this may reflect my own taste and relative expertise, it is also intentional. I reason that, if you have purchased an expensive cut of meat or seafood, you probably already know how to prepare it, or it is a special occasion that warrants figuring out how to do so properly. Similarly, I avoided getting too deeply into specific international cuisines (e.g., Asian, Indian). I included only recipes that could be made without visiting a specialty grocer in person or online. If you have an interest in, say, Thai cooking then you either already know more than I do and/or are going to look elsewhere to learn. I do include a few international recipes that use prepared sauces and/or spice blends that are widely available.

Sugar

Nutritional advice almost unanimously recommends minimizing (or even eliminating) the amount of sugar consumed. The obvious solution would be to simply skip all desserts, baked goods, pancakes, and other sweets. However, I think families can make great stride in reducing their total sugar intake by cutting soda, juice, candy, sweetened cereal and commercially prepared desserts. Since baked goods and desserts are some of the foods most likely to be ultra-processed, it makes sense to give you homemade options. These are often quite simple to make at home where you can control the ingredient quality, scale the recipe to your needs, and reduce the sugar content; significantly improving the nutritional profile while reducing cost.

You will notice that many of the savory recipes include small amounts of sugar or honey. When a recipe calls for just one to two teaspoons sugar, the sweetener is just to smooth out the flavor profile. Feel free to omit it or use a sugar substitute if you are taking a hard line on added sugars.

Using salt

You may also notice that most recipes here include only a small amount of salt or note salt as optional. I believe that using less salt lets the taste of high-quality ingredients shine through. However, this is a personal choice, and you may prefer to use more salt. (I will say that your taste will shift if you let it.) If you are considering increasing the salt in a recipe, don't forget that all canned and jarred ingredients already have salt, as well as any condiments and spice blends. However, here are some common rules of thumb for how much salt is typically recommended in cooking:

- Meat: 1 - 2 tsp per pound of raw meat
- Flour: ¼ - ½ tsp per cup of flour
- Grains/Cereals: ½ - 1 tsp per cup of water
- Pasta: 1 tsp per quart of water
- Soup: 1 tsp per quart

Real Food – Real Photos

Artistically stylized photos of food are lovely to look at, but you won't find them in this book. The photos accompanying the recipes here are pictures of Real Food, prepared according to the recipe in a normal home kitchen. No tricks, no special equipment, no exaggerated proportions: just the food as you can expect it to look when you prepare it at home. For example:

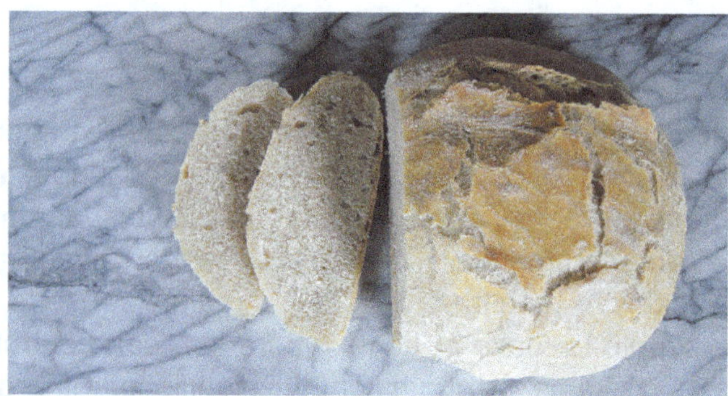

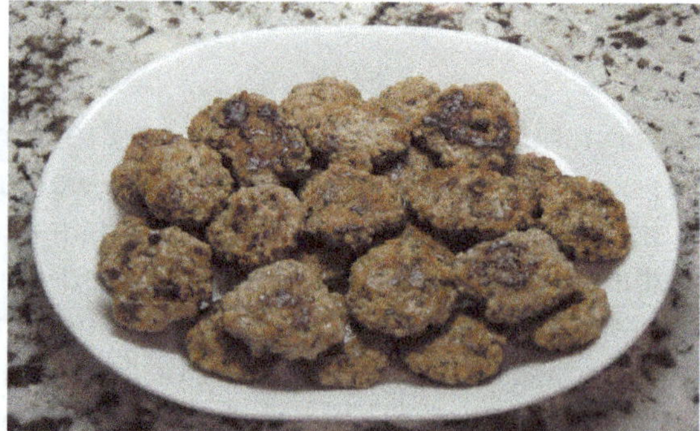

Vegetarian Dishes

You may notice that there are a lot of Agile Recipes™ in the "Veggie" category. Remember that this means that the recipe's major component is a "Veggie." This is just one more tool to help you manage your dietary goals; it does not mean that the dish is vegetarian.

Any recipe that is (or could be) vegetarian will have a superscript V at the end of the title. For example, the recipe for Cauliflower Marinara^{V} is both in the "Veggie" category and is a vegetarian dish. In this book, the vegetarian notation means that the recipe can be made without meat but there could be dairy products or eggs.

Agile Recipes™

There are 137 Agile Recipes™ (plus 144 additional listed recipe options) and simple-to-use charts with 40 recipes for marinades, salad dressings, and sauces in Chapter 4. They are organized by the type of dish to enable you to find the information you need as quickly and efficiently as possible.

For more information about Agile Recipes™ and to download PDF versions of all recipes please visit www.ReEngineeringtheKitchen.com.

Supporting Actors: Staples

It is easier to decide to cook when you are confident that you have all the ancillary ingredients on hand. You probably have a list of staples that you maintain automatically. However, I'd suggest you look at the list on the following page and evaluate if it makes sense for you to expand your list of staples. These are all items that can be stored for a long time so you will likely use them up eventually.

Suggested Essential Staples

Pantry	Fridge	Freezer	Spices
Baking Powder	BBQ Sauce	Butter	Basil
Baking Soda	Buttermilk Powder	Cream (for cooking)	Cardamon
Bouillon Powder *	Cream	Garlic *	Chili Powder
Breadcrumbs (Panko)	Curry Paste *	Ginger *	Cinnamon
Brown Sugar	Eggs	Milk (for cooking)	Cloves
Canola or Safflower Oil	Garlic – Minced Jar *	Nuts	Cumin
Coconut Oil	Ginger Paste *	OJ Concentrate	Curry *
Cooking Spray	Hot/Chili Sauce	Sour Cream (for cooking)	Dehydrated Onion
Corn Starch	Jam	Yogurt (for cooking)	Dill
Extra Virgin Olive Oil	Ketchup		Fennel Seeds
Flour	Lemon Juice		Garlic Powder
Honey	Mayonnaise		Ginger
Tomatoes and/or Sauce	Milk		Herbs de Provence
Tomato Paste – Can	Mustard – Dijon		Nutmeg
Vinegar – Apple Cider	Mustard – Yellow		Oregano
Vinegar – Balsamic	Onions		Paprika
Vinegar – White	Parmesan Cheese		Pepper
Vinegar – Wine	Sour Cream or Yogurt		Poultry Seasoning
White Sugar	Soy Sauce		Red Pepper Flakes
	Stock Paste *		Rosemary
	Syrup – Maple		Sage
	Tomato Paste – Tube		Salt
	Worcestershire Sauce		Thyme
			Vanilla
* Item is available in different formats; choose the one that you prefer.			

CHAPTER 4

AGILE RECIPES™

Any recipe that is or could be vegetarian has a superscript V at the end of the title.

BREAKFAST (CONT.)

DESSERT

DESSERT (CONT.)

MAIN

Main (cont.)

85 Baked Rice Casserole[V]
- Chicken Broccoli
- Chicken Pot Pie
- Savory Mushroom

86 Balsamic Glazed Chicken
87 Beef Stroganoff
88 Black Bean and Sweet Potato Chili[V]
89 Chicken Curry[V]
- Classic
- Vegetarian

90 Chicken Divan
91 Chicken Mushroom Marsala
92 Chicken Paillard
93 Chicken Paprika
94 Chicken Salad
- Deli Style
- Napa
- Cherry Chicken
- Waldorf Chicken

95 Chili Express
96 Citrus Grilled Shrimp
97 Crab Cakes
99 Enchilada Surprise[V]
- Chicken, Pork or Beef
- Vegetarian
- Tex-Mex

100 Fajitas
101 Fried Rice[V]
102 Hammered Chops

Main (cont.)

103 Italian Sausage – Scratch
104 Lasagna Florentine[V]
105 Lemon Butter Baked Fish
106 Lentils del Sol[V]
107 Marinated Flank Steak
108 Meatballs – Italian
109 Meatloaf
- Classic
- BBQ
- Italian
- Mushroom
- Cheeseburger

110 Oven-Fried Chicken
- Classic
- Gluten Free
- Italian
- Cajun

112 Palak Paneer[V]
113 Picadillo
114 Poached Chicken
115 Roast Pork Tenderloin
- Apple Cider Vinegar
- Dry Rub
- BBQ

116 Salmon with Sweet Mustard Glaze
- Citrus
- Blackened

117 Shrimp & Cheesy Grits
118 Shrimp Scampi

MAIN (CONT.)

MARINADES & BRINES

SALADS

SALAD DRESSINGS

SALAD DRESSINGS (CONT.)

SAUCES

SAUCES (CONT.)

SIDES

SIDES (CONT.)

SIDES (CONT.)

SOUP

PROTEIN OTHER	**Baked Salsa Dip**^{V} **Makes about 1 cup**	**Appetizer**
INGREDIENTS		**SUBSTITUTE**
1	Jar of salsa, 16 oz	
8 oz	Goat cheese log	
STEPS		
1	Preheat oven to 350°F.	
2	Cut goat cheese log into disks about 1 inch thick. Arrange in the bottom of a shallow baking dish or pan (at least 1 quart).	
3	Pour salsa over the cheese.	
4	Bake until golden on top and bubbly, about 35-45 minutes.	
5	Serve with bread, chips, or crackers.	

PROTEIN OTHER	**Hummus**^{V} **Makes about 1 cup**	**Appetizer**
INGREDIENTS		**SUBSTITUTE**
1	15.5 oz can chickpeas (~2 C), drained	Any canned or cooked white beans
3 Tbsp	Extra Virgin Olive Oil	
2 Tbsp	Lemon juice - fresh	Any lemon juice
1-2 cloves	Garlic	Jarred minced garlic or garlic powder
½ tsp	Salt	
¼ tsp	Ground cumin	
2 Tbsp	Tahini (optional)	
2-4 Tbsp	Water - just enough so that mixture will blend	
STEPS		
1	Combine all ingredients including 2 Tbsp of water in blender, food processor or immersion blender cup.	
2	Blend until the mixture is a smooth texture. Add water in 1 tsp increments if necessary.	
3	Serve with a spinkle of paprika on top. Great with any flat bread, crackers, or raw veggies.	

PROTEIN MEAT	**Buffalo Chicken Dip** **Makes about 5 cups**	**Appetizer**
INGREDIENTS		**SUBSTITUTE**
2	12.5 oz cans Chunk Chicken Breast	3 C shredded cooked chicken
4 oz	Cream cheese, room temperature	Low fat or fat free cream cheese
1 C	Greek yogurt, plain	Full fat or non-fat
1 C	Shredded mozzarella cheese	
½ C	Crumbled blue cheese or Gorgonzola	Light blue cheese
½ C	Hot sauce (Frank's or other)	⅓ C for a less spicy result
STEPS		
1	Preheat oven to 350°F. Grease a shallow (1½ - 2 qt) baking dish.	
2	Drain the canned chicken and shred the meat.	
3	Mix all of the ingredients in a bowl and stir until everything is well incorporated.	
4	Pour into the prepared baking dish. (At this point it may be refrigerated for 24 hours.)	
5	Bake for 30-40 minutes or until the cheese is melted and bubbly, and starting to crisp along the edges.	
6	Serve with corn tortilla chips, celery sticks, crackers, or bread.	

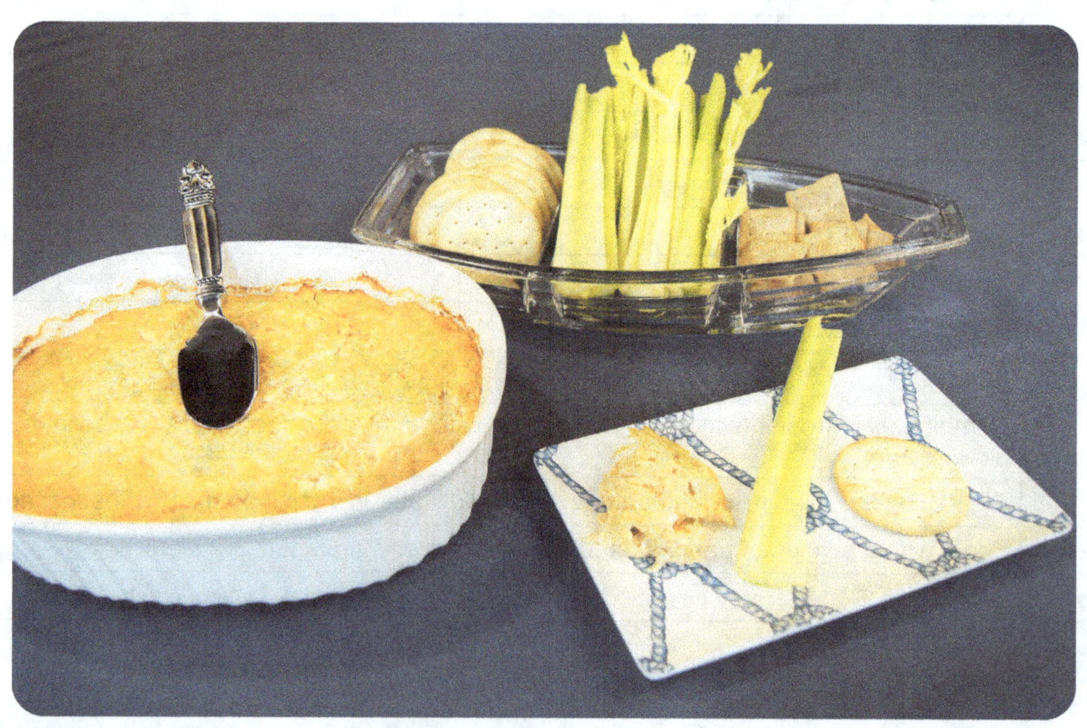

PROTEIN OTHER	Cheese Fondue^V Makes about 2 cups	Appetizer
INGREDIENTS		**SUBSTITUTE**
1 Tbsp	Corn starch	
1 C	White wine - cool	
2 C	Swiss or Gruyere cheese - grated (8 oz)	
STEPS		
1	Measure cold wine into saucepan and stir in corn starch until well mixed.	
2	Warm the corn starch and wine mixture over medium heat, stirring until thickened. Do not allow to boil.	
3	Add the grated cheese to the thickened sauce and stir over low heat until cheese melts.	
4	Return to heat only as necessary to fully incorporate and/or to warm.	
5	Garnish with parsley, if desired.	
6	Serve in a fondue pot, a small crock pot, or a ceramic baking dish which has been pre-warmed. Serve with chunks of bread, sliced apples, or veggies to be dipped in the fondue.	

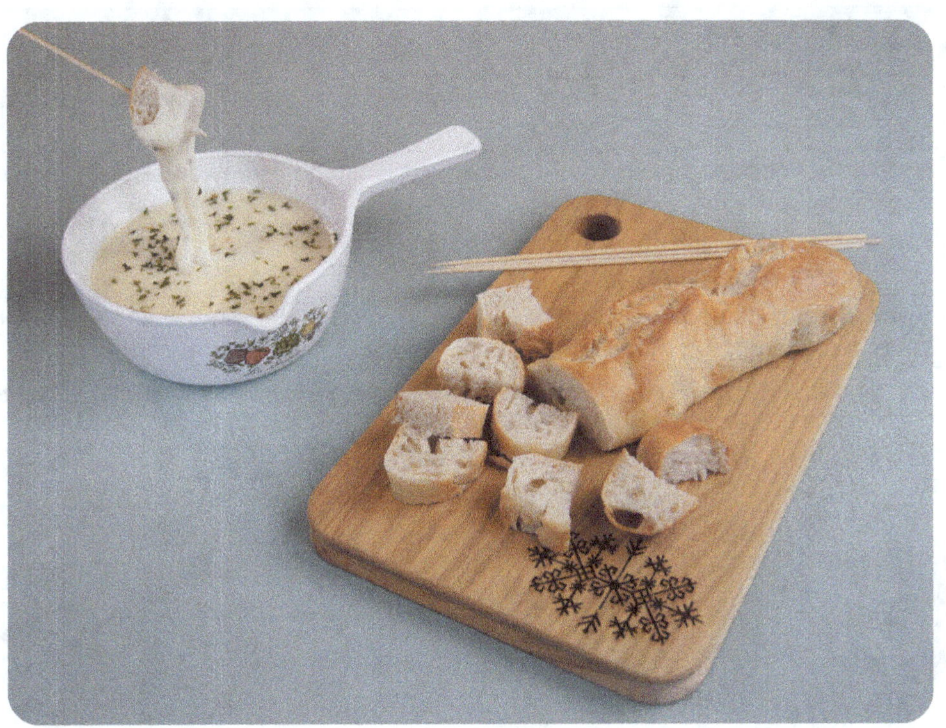

PROTEIN OTHER	**Crispy Chickpea Snacks[V]** **Makes 3 cups**	**Appetizer**
INGREDIENTS		**SUBSTITUTE**
2	15.5 oz cans chickpeas, drained	
1 Tbsp	Extra Virgin Olive Oil	Any olive oil, avocado oil or any other neutral cooking oil
1 tsp	Salt	
½ tsp	Cracked black pepper	Other spices - see options below
STEPS		
1	Preheat oven to 375°F.	
2	Rinse chickpeas and dry well by rubbing between paper towels. Remove any skins that have come loose in the drying.	
3	Spread dry chickpeas on a rimmed baking sheet lined with parchment paper.	
4	Bake for 35 minutes until chickpeas are crispy but still a bit soft in the middle. Shake the pan a few times during cooking.	
5	Remove from oven, put chickpeas into a bowl and toss with oil, salt and spices. Return to sheet pan and roast for another 10 minutes until crispy but not burnt.	
6	Remove from oven and allow to cool. Store loosely covered.	
OPTIONS		
A	**Spicy**: Replace black pepper with 1 tsp each of chili powder, cumin and paprika. Add ¼ tsp cayenne for an extra kick.	
B	**Herb-y**: In addition to black pepper, toss with ¼ tsp garlic powder and 2 tsp thyme, Italian seasoning or oregano.	
C	**Sweet**: Cut salt in half and replace black pepper with 1 Tbsp brown sugar and 2 tsp cinnamon or pumpkin pie spice.	
D	**Spice Blend**: Replace pepper with 2-3 tsp of your favorite prepared spice blend, e.g. Chili-Lime, Seasoning Salt, Adobe, Cajun, etc. Omit salt if your blend contains salt.	

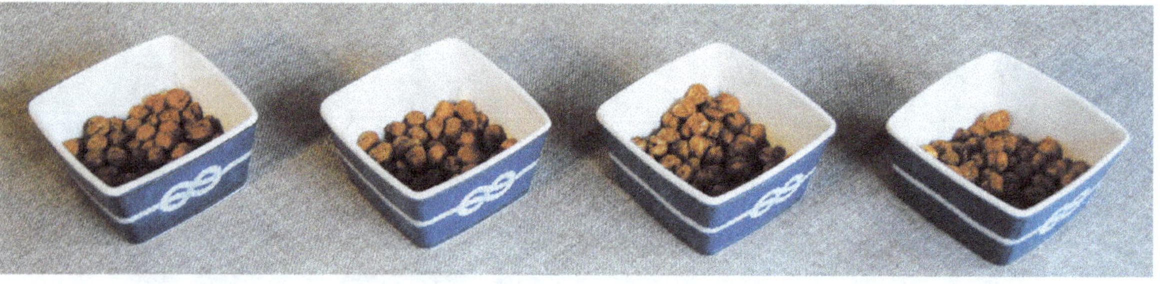

VEGGIE	**Guacamole Fresca^{V}** **Makes about 2 cups**	**Appetizer**
INGREDIENTS		**SUBSTITUTE**
2	Avocados, Haas, ripe	4 mini avocados
2 Tbsp	Fresh orange juice	1 Tbsp lime or lemon juice, or orange juice concentrate
½	Red onion, small, diced	White or sweet onion
½ tsp	Minced garlic	¼ tsp garlic granules
1	Medium tomato	
½ Tbsp	Jalapeno pepper, finely diced (optional)	
4 Tbsp	Cilantro, coarsley chopped (optional)	
	Salt to taste	
STEPS		
1	Cut avocados in half, remove pit and then slice into cubes. Scoop avocado out of shell into mixing bowl. Leave in cubes if you want a chunky end product or mash for smooth.	
2	Add the orange juice (or other citrus juice) to the avocado and turn to coat.	
3	Cut the tomato and remove most of the seeds and surrounding gel. Dice the tomato.	
4	Add the garlic, onion, tomato, pepper, and cilantro (if using) to the avocados and mix well.	
5	Add salt to taste. Cover with plastic wrap against surface and refrigerate if you are not using immediately.	
6	Serve with corn chips or with any Mexican dish.	

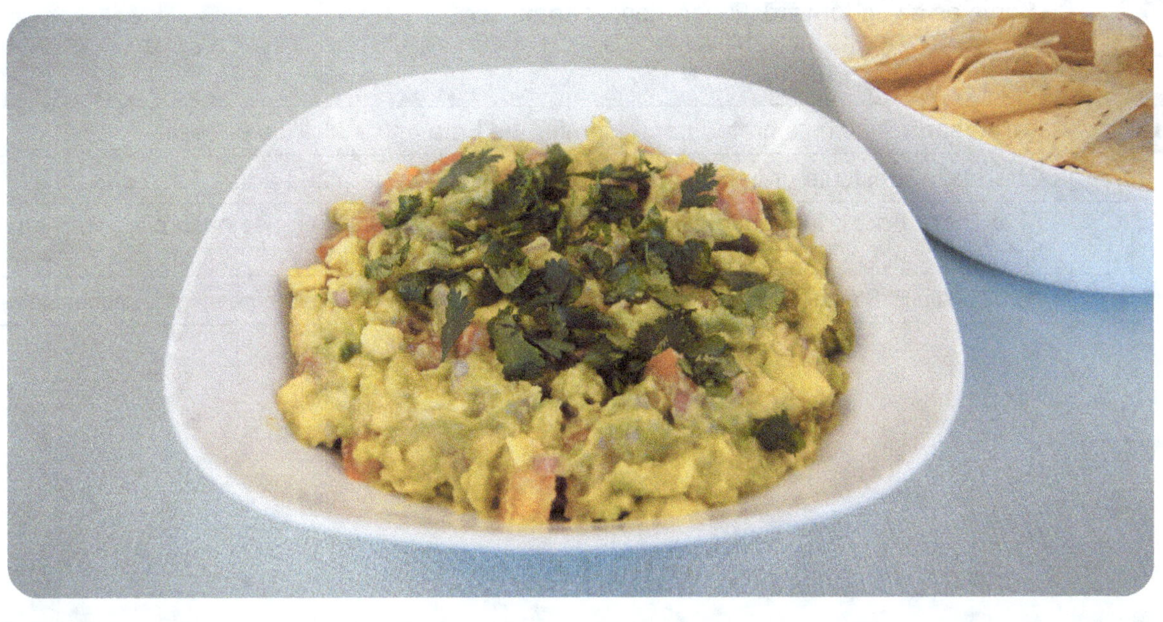

VEGGIE	**Spinach Bites**[V] **Makes 24 one-inch bites**	**Appetizer**
INGREDIENTS		**SUBSTITUTE**
16 oz	Frozen chopped spinach	
1 C	Crumbled Feta cheese	
2	Eggs, large or larger	
2 Tbsp	Butter	Olive oil
1 tsp	Minced garlic	¼ tsp garlic powder
½ tsp	Dehydrated onion flakes	¼ tsp onion powder
½ C	Flour	¼ C corn starch
1 tsp	Salt	
1 tsp	Baking powder	
STEPS		
1	Preheat oven to 375°F. Prepare baking sheet by lining it with parchment paper. Alternatively, oil the bottoms of a non-stick mini-muffin tin.	
2	Cook spinach in covered microwave-safe dish for 7 minutes on high. Drain well and squeeze out excess water. A mesh strainer works well. Add butter to warm spinach.	
3	Combine eggs, cheese and spices then mix well. Stir in the cooked spinach	
4	Add flour, salt and baking powder to the egg/spinach mixture and stir well. At this point, the mixture may be refrigerated for a day before baking.	
5	Scoop about 2 Tbsp of mixture at a time onto the baking sheet or into the muffin tins. A 1½" cookie dough scoop works well. Spritz tops with olive oil if desired.	
6	Bake for 20 minutes. Should be crisp on the outside and at least 160° F on the inside.	
7	Serve as a veg-forward, finger-friendly appetizer,	
OPTIONS		
A	**Parmesan:** Substitute grated parmesan for the Feta and add 1 tsp of basil.	
B	**Cheddar:** Substitute grated aged sharp cheddar for the feta and add 1 Tbsp of parsley.	
C	**Side Dish:** For an interesting way to serve spinach, plate several spinach bites with an entrée. For larger bites (4 Tbsp), cook an additional 5 minutes.	

Photo on page 52

MEASUREMENTS CONVERSIONS

• COOKING - BAKING •

CUP	ONCES	MILLILITERS	TBSP.
1/16	1/2 oz	15 ml	1
1/8	1 oz	30 ml	3
1/4	2 oz	59 ml	4
1/3	2.5 oz	79 ml	5.5
3/8	3 oz	90 ml	6
1/2	4 oz	118 ml	8
2/3	5 oz	158 ml	11
3/4	6 oz	177 ml	12
1	8 oz	240 ml	16

GRAIN	Banana Bread[V] Makes 2 loaves	Bread
INGREDIENTS		**SUBSTITUTE**
8 Tbsp	Butter, melted	Margarine
¾ C	Sugar	Brown sugar or dry artificial sweetener
3	Eggs, large or XL	
½ C	Milk	Cream or Half & Half or half cream/half water
4-5	Bananas, ripe and smashed	
2 C	Flour (240 g)	Substitute up to half whole wheat flour
1 Tbsp	Baking soda	
1 tsp	Baking powder	
¼ tsp	Salt (optional)	
STEPS		
1	Preheat oven to 350°F or 325°F if using glass loaf pans.	
2	In a large mixing bowl, mix bananas, eggs, milk, and sugar together well.	
3	Add dry ingredients to banana mixture and mix well.	
4	Stir in melted butter.	
5	Pour batter into two 8 inch greased loaf pans.	
6	Bake for 40-60 minutes. Center will become firm. Test for doneness by inserting knife near the center; knife will not be clean, but should not be gooey.	
7	Store covered or wrapped in foil. Freezes well.	
OPTIONS		
A	Stir ½ C chopped nuts or ½ C chocolate into batter.	
B	If using a muffin pan or larger loaf pans, start checking for doneness after 30 minutes.	

Photo on page 52

GRAIN	Beer Bread[V] Makes 1 loaf	Bread
INGREDIENTS		**SUBSTITUTE**
3 C	Flour (360 g), up to 1/3 whole wheat	Self rising flour - omit baking powder and salt
1½ Tbsp	Baking powder	
1½ tsp	Salt	
2 Tbsp	Sugar or honey	Up to ¼ C
¼ C	Butter, melted	2 Tbsp more for top crust, optional
12 oz	Beer, any type	
STEPS		
1	Preheat oven to 350°F. Coat inside of 8" x 4" loaf pan with oil.	
2	Mix dry ingredients together in large bowl.	
3	Stir beer and melted butter into dry ingredients. Mix only enough to combine.	
4	Pour into loaf pan. Pour additional 2 Tbsp melted butter on top if desired.	
5	Bake for about one hour. Start checking for doneness after 45 minutes; center will spring back when pressed and toothpick or knife will come out clean.	
6	Serve with butter, cheese, soup, or stew. Great option to stretch a meal on short notice. Warm bread is a welcome addition to any appetizer tray.	

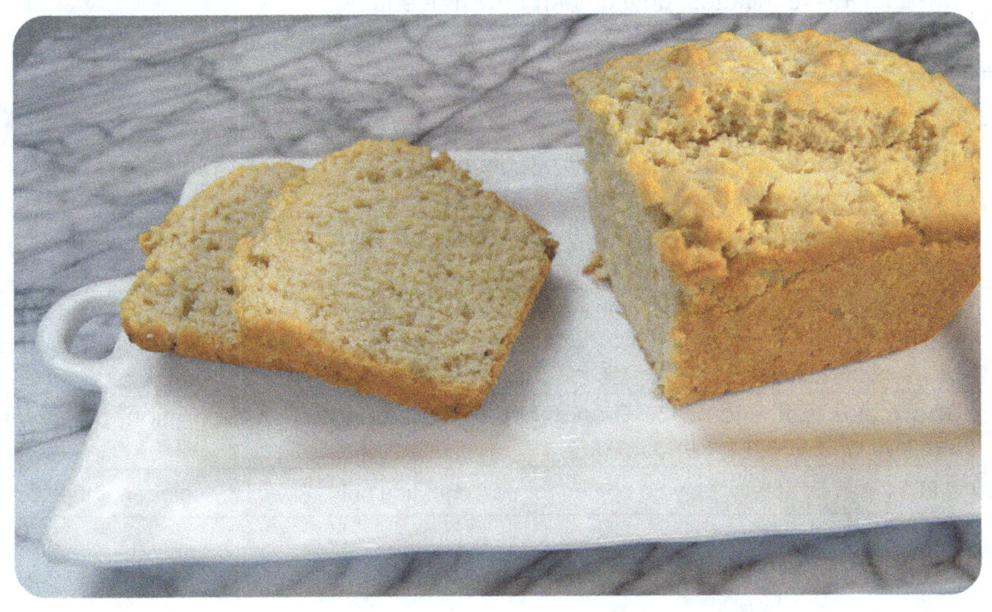

GRAIN	Biscuit/Shortcake[V] Makes 6 biscuits	Bread
INGREDIENTS		**SUBSTITUTE**
3 Tbsp	Butter	Crisco or margarine
1½ C	Flour (180 g)	1 C rice flour + ½ C tapioca flour (GF) or substitute up to 50% whole grain flour
½ Tbsp	Baking powder	
½ Tbsp	Sugar	Brown sugar or dry sugar substitute
½ tsp	Salt	
½ C	Milk	Half & Half or buttermilk or half cream/half water
STEPS		
1	Preheat oven to 400°F. Grease pan or line with parchment paper.	
2	In a heat-proof glass bowl or 4 C glass measuring cup, warm butter to room temp in micro.	
3	Add flour to bowl with butter. If you have a scale, weigh flour directly into your bowl.	
4	Add baking powder, salt, and sugar to flour. Stir to distribute dry ingredients.	
5	With a fork, work the flour mixture and butter together until it becomes coarse and dry.	
6	Add milk and stir just enough to fully incorporate.	
7	Use scoop or spoon to make six rounded biscuits. Each should be about 1½ inches high.	
8	Bake for 12-18 minutes, until golden brown at edges.	
9	Store covered. May reheat for 5 minutes in 350°F oven or 15 seconds in micro.	
OPTIONS		
A	**Rolled Biscuits:** Roll dough on floured surface to about ¾ inch thickness. Cut with cookie cutter or with a glass or jar of desired diameter.	
B	**Cheese Biscuits:** Stir in ½ C any shredded cheese into dough. Can add ½ tsp garlic powder to dry ingredients for more savory flavor.	
C	**Cinnamon Bun Biscuits:** Place biscuits close together in 9 inch pan, flatten each slightly by hand. Mix 2 Tbsp soft butter with 1 tsp cinnamon and 2 Tbsp sugar. Spread paste over biscuits prior to baking.	
D	**Shortcake:** Add another ½ Tbsp of sugar to the dough. For decoration, brush with butter and sprinkle with sugar prior to baking.	

GRAIN	Corn Bread[V] Makes one 9 inch pan	Bread
INGREDIENTS		**SUBSTITUTE**
1¼ C	All purpose flour (150 g)	
¾ C	Corn meal	
1 Tbsp	Baking powder	
½ tsp	Salt	
4 Tbsp	Sugar, white	
1	Egg, large or XL, beaten	
3 Tbsp	Butter, melted	
1 C	Milk	
1 C	Corn, cooked and well drained (optional)	Fresh, canned or frozen
STEPS		
1	Preheat oven to 400°F.	
2	Prepare baking pan. Can use well oiled cast iron skillet, cake pan or pie pan.	
3	In a large bowl mix together flour, corn meal, baking powder, salt and sugar.	
4	Add milk, egg, and melted butter to bowl and mix. Fold in corn if using.	
5	Pour batter into pan and bake for 30-40 minutes, until golden. A toothpick inserted in the center should come out clean.	

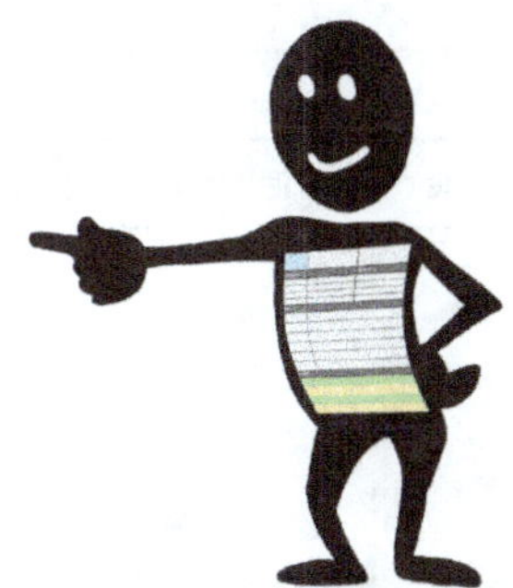

Scoop Biscuits

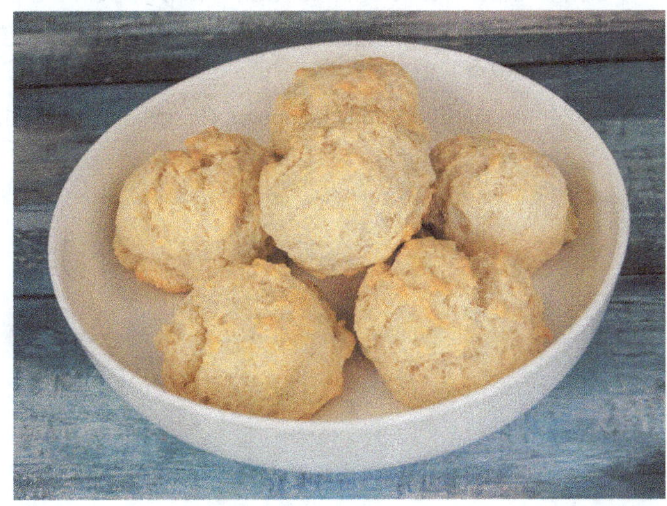

GRAIN	**Irish Soda Bread**[V] **Makes 1 loaf**	**Bread**
INGREDIENTS		**SUBSTITUTE**
4 C	All purpose flour (480 g)	Up to ⅓ whole wheat
1 tsp	Baking powder	
1 tsp	Baking soda	
½ tsp	Salt	
2 Tbsp	Sugar, white or brown	Up to ¼ C
1	Egg, large or XL	
4 Tbsp	Butter, room temperature	
1½ C	Buttermilk	1½ Tbsp vinegar + 11 oz Milk
1 C	Raisins (optional)	
STEPS		
1	Preheat oven to 375°F.	
2	Prepare baking pan. Can use seasoned cast iron skillet or dutch oven. A baking sheet or cake pan can be oiled or lined with parchment paper.	
3	In a large bowl mix together flour, baking powder, baking soda, salt and sugar.	
4	Work butter into the flour mixture with pastry cutter, fork or fingers until crumbly.	
5	Beat buttermilk and egg together then pour into flour mixture. Add raisins if using.	
6	Stir until no dry flour remains. If dough is too sticky, add a little bit of flour. Knead dough about eight times.	
7	Form a round loaf with the dough and place on the prepared pan. Cut a shallow X across the top surface of the dough to ensure the loaf bakes evenly.	
8	Bake for 40-50 minutes.	

GRAIN	No Touch Bread[V] Makes one 1½ lb loaf	Bread
INGREDIENTS		**SUBSTITUTE**
4 C	Flour, all purpose (480 g)	Bread flour
2¼ tsp	Instant yeast (1 packet)	Active dry yeast
1 tsp	Kosher salt	
1⅔ C	Warm water (105-115°F)	
STEPS		
1	In a large bowl, mix the flour, salt and yeast. Add the warm water and mix. The temperature of the water should feel slightly hot, but not scalding.	
2	Mix until all of the flour is incorporated with spatula or spoon - silicone is best as the dough will not stick to it. Dough should be soft and sticky.	
3	Cover the bowl and allow dough to rise in a warm, but not hot, place. Dough should double in bulk in 1-2 hours.	
4	OPTIONAL STEP: When the dough has risen, you can refrigerate the dough for up to 2 days to allow the flavor to develop further. Allow the dough to warm up prior to next step.	
5	Preheat the oven to 450°F. Put your covered baking pan (Dutch oven or roasting pan with lid) in to preheat with the oven.	
6	Scrape from sides and fold the dough a few times forming a round loaf in the bowl. A silicone spatula is best, but you can use floured hands.	
7	Turn loaf onto a large sheet of parchment paper dusted with flour. Cover dough with the overturned bowl and allow to rise for 30 minutes.	
8	Using the parchment paper, lift loaf into the pre-heated covered pan and replace lid.	
9	Bake for 30 minutes with lid on. Remove lid and continue baking for an addition 10-15 minutes or until bread is done (internal temperature of about 200°F).	
10	Lift loaf out of pan with paper and allow to cool before slicing.	

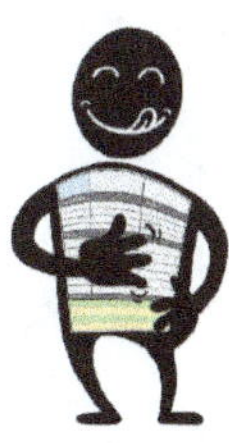

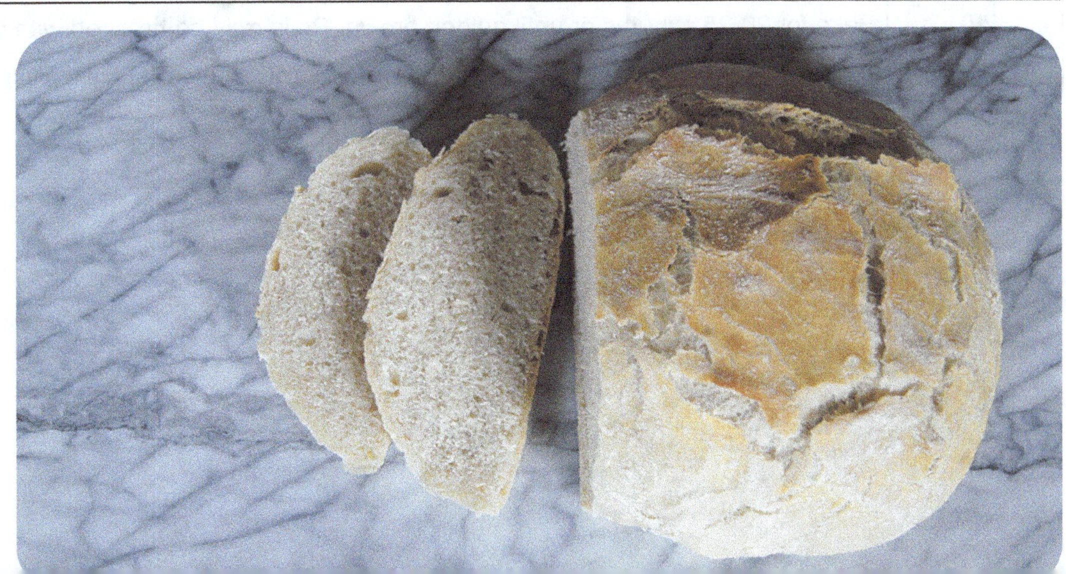

GRAIN	Yeast Rolls^{V} Makes 24 dinner rolls	Bread
INGREDIENTS		**SUBSTITUTE**
1 C	Milk	
½ C	Butter	Margarine
4 Tbsp	Sugar	
1 tsp	Salt	
1	Package active dry yeast (2¼ tsp)	Rapid rise yeast
2	Eggs, large or XL	
4 C	Flour, all purpose (480 g)	

STEPS	
1	Preheat oven to 375°F. Prepare a 9”x13” pan by coating with cooking spray. Can use two 8”x8” baking pans.
2	Scald milk in a large pan. Add butter, sugar and salt and allow to cool to lukewarm (110-115°F).
3	Mix in yeast and eggs with mixer or whisk.
4	Mix half the flour into the liquid with a whisk or mixer. Mix in the remaining flour with a spoon or spatula (silicone works well as the dough sticks less).
5	Turn dough onto floured surface and knead only until dough becomes smooth and elastic. Avoid adding more flour than necessary for handling.
6	Cover the dough and put in a warm place. Allow to rise until doubled in bulk, about 1 hour.
7	Punch down the dough to release the gas. Dough may be refrigerated at this point for up to 24 hours.
8	Divide the dough into 24 pieces, shaping each into a ball. Arrange dough balls in the pan(s).
9	Cover the dough with a clean towel and allow to rise in a warm place for about 1 hour. Dough should double in size.
10	Bake for 20-25 minutes or until golden brown. Rolls may be brushed with melted butter.

PROTEIN MEAT	**Biscuits and Gravy** **Serves 4-6**	**Breakfast**
INGREDIENTS		**SUBSTITUTE**
3 Tbsp	Butter	Any oil or rendered meat fat.
2 Tbsp	Flour	
2 C	Milk	
1 lb	Pork breakfast sausage, browned & drained	
	Salt, pepper, and red pepper flakes to taste	
STEPS		
1	Make 12 biscuits per the Biscuit/Shortcake recipe on page 44 (a double recipe).	
2	Melt butter in small pan. Add flour.	
3	Cook flour and butter over medium low heat for at least three minutes. Should gently bubble.	
4	Remove pan from heat to cool slightly. Add all of the liquid, stirring to fully incorporate.	
5	Return pan to medium low heat, stirring constantly until the sauce thickens. Do not allow to come to a boil. Remove from heat when thickened.	
6	Stir in the browned & drained sausage.	
7	Add seasonings to the sauce. Return to low heat only as necessary to fully incorporate and warm.	
8	Serve the gravy over the fresh biscuits.	
OPTIONS		
A	**Sweet Version:** Use 1 lb sweet Italian sauage, cooked and drained, in place of the pork breakfast sausage.	

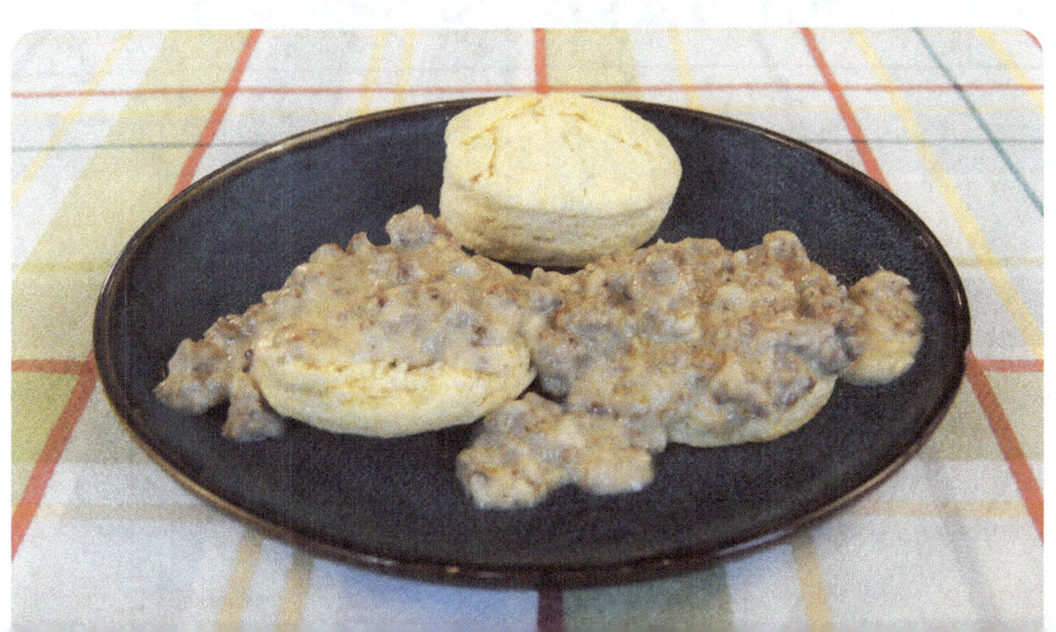

PROTEIN MEAT	**Breakfast Sausage** **Makes 8 patties**	**Breakfast**
INGREDIENTS		**SUBSTITUTE**
1 lb	Ground pork	Ground turkey or chicken
2 tsp	Sage, ground	
2 tsp	Thyme	
1 tsp	Fennel seed, ground	
1 tsp	Salt	
¾ tsp	Black pepper, ground	
½ tsp	Red pepper flakes (optional)	
⅛ tsp	Nutmeg, ground	
STEPS		
1	Mix meat with all spices until thoroughly incorporated. Best if allowed to rest for 4-24 hours in refrigerator, but may be used immediately.	
2	Shape into patties, if desired.	
3	Fry with a little oil if needed. Sausage made with turkey will be drier and need oil to brown nicely.	

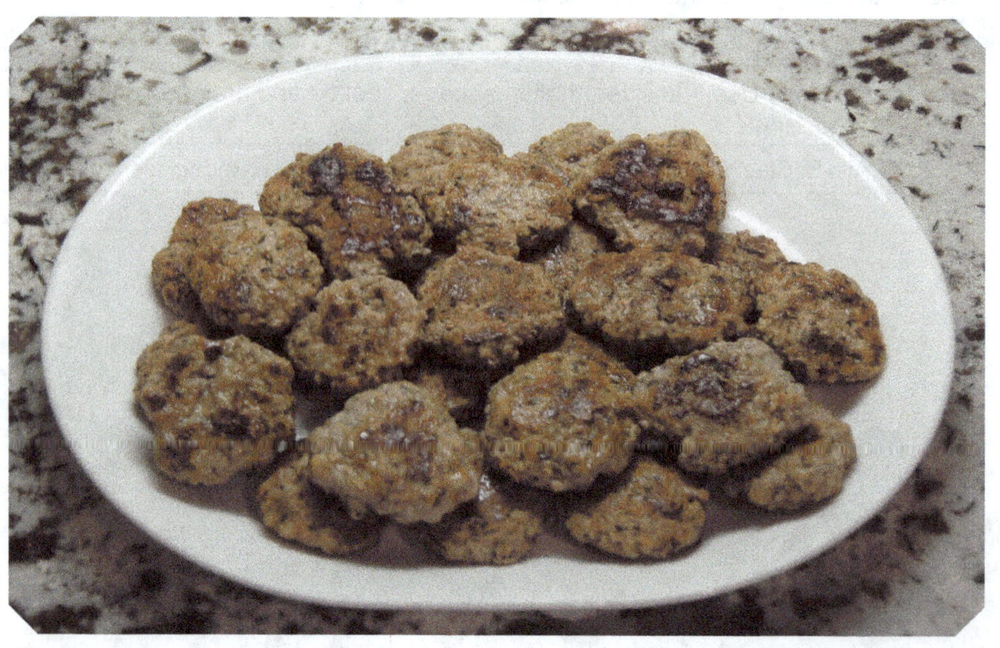

PROTEIN OTHER	**Egg Cups^{V}** **Makes 12 cups**	**Breakfast**
INGREDIENTS		**SUBSTITUTE**
8	Eggs, large or XL	
1 C	Cottage cheese	
1½ tsp	Corn starch	
¼ C	Bacon, cooked and diced (optional)	Sausage, pancetta, diced onion or pepper
6 oz	Shredded cheese	
½ tsp	Black pepper	
½ tsp	Salt	
½ tsp	Onion flakes or red pepper flakes (optional)	

STEPS	
1	Preheat oven to 325°F. On lower oven rack, place a pan with 1 inch of hot water in it. This step is not essential, but the humidity keeps the eggs from drying out.
2	Spray muffin tin with cooking spray.
3	Brown and dice the bacon or other meat if using.
4	Combine the eggs, cottage cheese, corn starch and spices together, mixing well. Best done in a blender or mixer, but can use a bowl, and whisk vigorously.
5	In each muffin tin, put 1 tsp of bacon, ½ oz shredded cheese.
6	Pour egg mixture into tins and fill almost to the top, about ¼ C each. If there is a little extra egg mixture, it can be baked in either silicone cups or custard cups.
7	Bake for 25 minutes or until eggs are cooked. A knife inserted should come out clean.
8	Serve warm. Extras freeze well.

OPTIONS	
A	**Ham & Swiss**: Use finely diced ham instead of bacon and shredded Swiss or Gruyere cheese.
B	**Veggie**: Replace bacon with finely diced onion and red pepper. Start with ½ C veggies and put 2 tsp in each cup.
C	**Sausage & Cheddar**: Replace bacon with cooked sausage crumbles and use a sharp shredded cheddar cheese.
D	**Greek**: Replace bacon with ½ C cooked and well drained spinach. Use 2 tsp spinach per tin. Replace shredded cheese with crumbled feta.

Photo on page 52

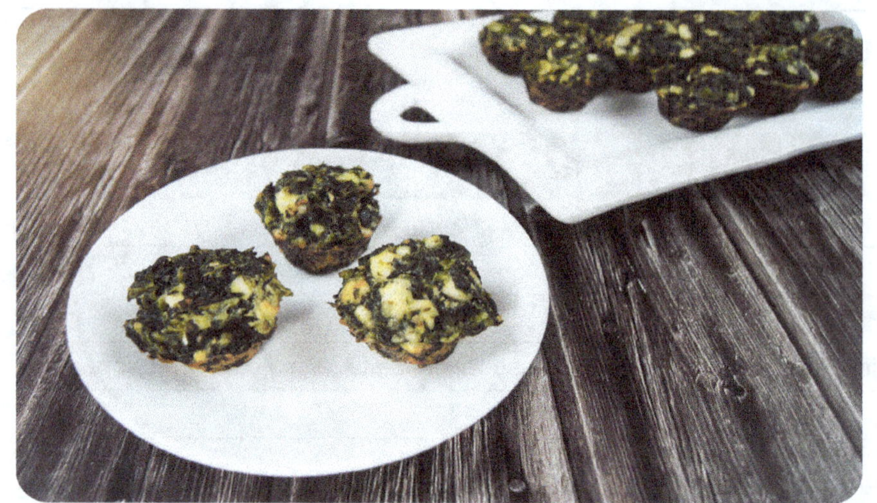

Spinach Bites

Recipe on page 40

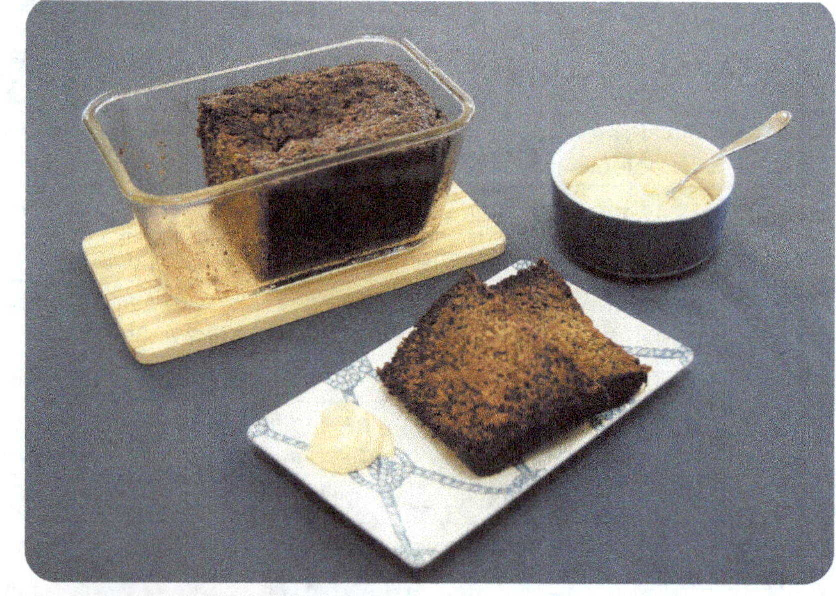

Banana Bread

Recipe on page 42

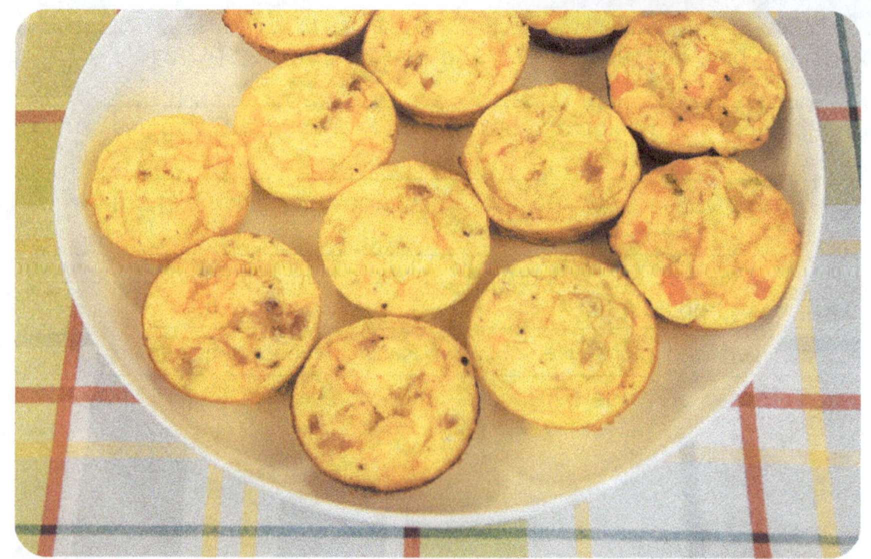

Egg Cups

Recipe on page 51

PROTEIN OTHER	**French Toast Casserole**[V] **Makes 6-10 servings**	**Breakfast**
INGREDIENTS		**SUBSTITUTE**
12 oz	Bread, cubed or torn into chunks	Buns, rolls, or bagels
¾ C	Milk	
1 C	Cottage cheese	Ricotta cheese
3	Eggs, large or XL	
¼ C	Sugar, white	Brown sugar, honey, or sugar substitute
1 tsp	Vanilla extract	Lemon extract
2 C	Berries, fresh	Frozen berries, thawed and drained
STEPS		
1	Preheat oven to 350°F. Generously grease a 9 x 13 inch pan or 2½ quart casserole dish.	
2	Put bread in a large bowl and pour milk over it. If your bread is dry, add another ¼ C of milk. Stir and allow all milk to soak in.	
3	In a separate small bowl, add cottage cheese, eggs, sugar, and vanilla. Beat well - an immersion blender is ideal, but can be whisked vigorously by hand.	
4	Pour cottage cheese and egg mixture over bread and stir to incorporate.	
5	Gently fold berries into bread/cheese/egg mixture and pour into baking pan.	
6	Bake for 35-45 minutes, until top is golden and center is firm.	
7	Serve with syrup, powdered sugar, or whipped cream.	

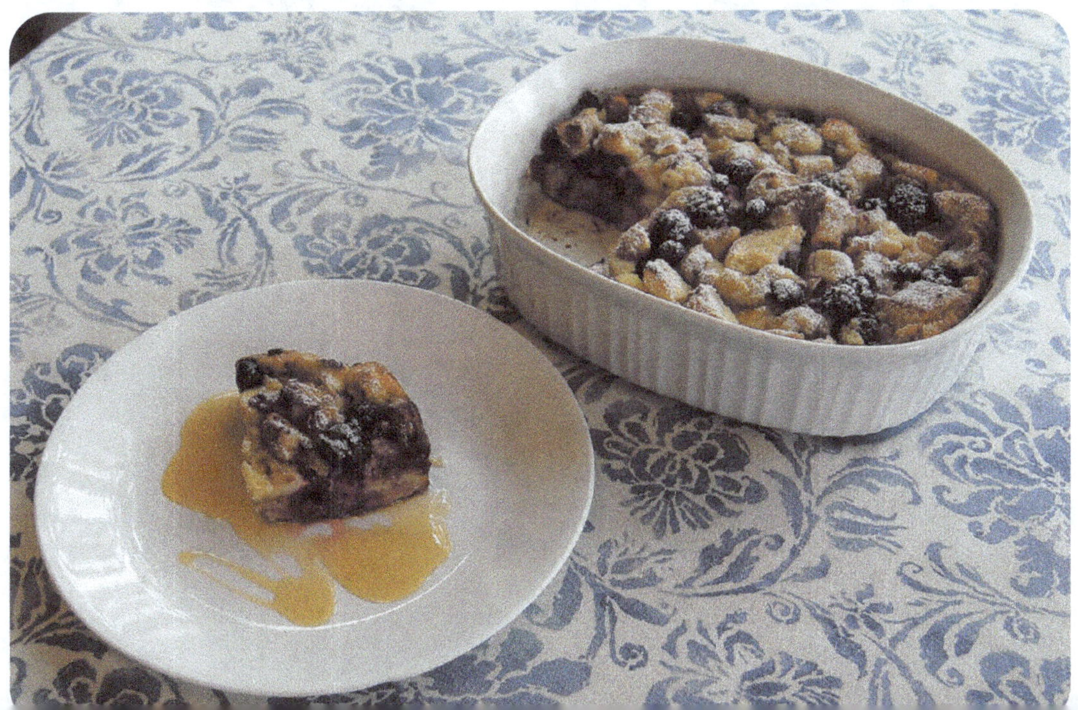

GRAIN	Oatmeal Pancakes[V] Serves 2-3	Breakfast
INGREDIENTS		**SUBSTITUTE**
1 C	Flour (120 g)	Up to ⅓ whole wheat
¾ C	Oats, Old Fashioned	Quick oats
1 tsp	Baking powder	
¼ C	Brown sugar	White sugar
¼ tsp	Salt	
1 C	Milk	½ C cream + ½ C water
1	Egg, large or XL	
1 Tbsp	Oil	Melted butter
STEPS		
1	In a large bowl, mix all dry ingredients.	
2	Beat milk, egg and oil together then add to dry ingredients. Mix well.	
3	Allow to stand 5-10 minutes.	
4	Cook batter ¼ to ½ cup at a time in a medium hot pan or griddle that has been lightly oiled.	
5	Makes 2 cups batter, approximately 8 four inch diameter pancakes.	

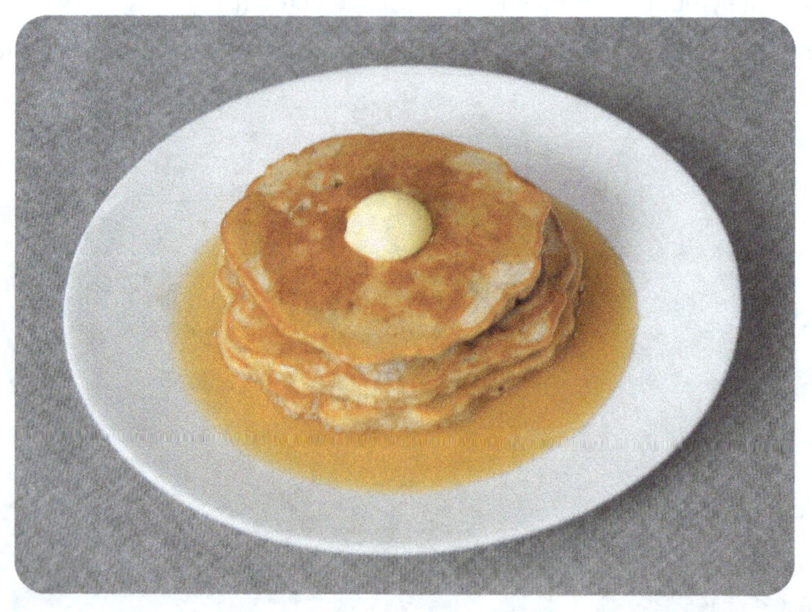

PROTEIN OTHER	**Potato Frittata[V]** **Serves 6**	**Breakfast**
INGREDIENTS		**SUBSTITUTE**
8	Eggs, large or XL	
2	Potatoes, medium (approx. 1 lb)	Leftover potatoes
1	Medium onion, sliced thinly	
2 Tbsp	Extra Virgin Olive Oil	
¼ C	Milk	Cream
½ tsp	Salt	
¼ tsp	Cracked black pepper	
STEPS		
1	Preheat oven to 350°F.	
2	Cook potatoes to tender by either boiling in water or microwaving. Can use leftover potatoes. Cut potatoes into slices or cubes no thicker than ¼ inch.	
3	In a large (12 inch) oven-proof skillet, sauté onion until soft. Add potatoes and brown slightly. Distribute onions and potatoes evenly in pan.	
4	In a bowl, whip eggs, milk, salt and pepper together.	
5	Pour egg mixture over onions and potatoes, spreading evenly.	
6	Bake in oven for 20-25 minutes, until eggs are set.	
7	Serve warm or room temperature.	
OPTIONS		
A	**Bacon & Cheddar**: Fry 3 strips of diced bacon in pan. Omit olive oil. Use the residual bacon fat to saute onions and potatoes. Add ½ C shredded cheddar cheese into egg mixture.	
B	**Veggie**: Increase the vegetable content by adding up to ½ C chopped bell peppers, spinach, or asparagas. If you add more than ½ C, decrease onion or potato proportionately.	
C	**Pasta**: Replace potatoes with 2 C cooked pasta. Stir ½ C Parmesan cheese into egg mixture.	

Photo on page 65

PROTEIN OTHER	**Ricotta Pancakes**[V] **Makes ~ twelve 5" pancakes**	**Breakfast**
INGREDIENTS		**SUBSTITUTE**
4	Eggs, large or XL	
1 tsp	Vanilla extract	
¼ C	Sugar	
1 C	Milk	
1 C	Ricotta cheese	Cottage cheese
1½ C	Flour (180 g)	
3 Tbsp	Butter, melted	
STEPS		
1	Whisk egg, vanilla and sugar together.	
2	Add milk and ricotta cheese, mixing well. If using cottage cheese, use an immersion blender to fully mix.	
3	Add flour and baking powder and whisk until smooth.	
4	Pour in melted butter slowly while continuing to stir.	
5	Preheat sauté pan lightly coated with oil over medium heat. The pan is hot enough when a drop of water will "dance" but oil is not smoking.	
6	Pour about ⅓ C batter into hot pan, spreading batter if necessary so that it is not too thick.	
7	Cook until the pancake is set, then flip to cook an additional couple minutes.	
8	Serve with your favorite topping: fruit and whipped cream, syrup, jam, chocolate-hazelnut spread, powdered sugar.	

PROTEIN MEAT	**Sausage Brunch Bake** **Makes 8-10 servings**	**Breakfast**
INGREDIENTS		**SUBSTITUTE**
1 lb	Pork breakfast sausage	Turkey breakfast sausage
9	Eggs, large or XL	
1 C	Milk	
12 oz	Co-Jack cheese, shredded	Any mild cheese or cheese blend
8 oz	Bread, in 1 inch cubes or chunks	Any type of yeast bread or roll
½ tsp	Salt and pepper, each	
STEPS		
1	Preheat oven to 350°F and prepare 9 x 9 inch (or 2½ quart) baking dish by coating interior of pan with oil.	
2	Brown sausage and then drain well.	
3	In a bowl, whisk eggs, salt, pepper, and milk together.	
4	Put bread, sausage crumbles and half of the cheese in the pan.	
5	Pour egg and milk mixture over the bread in the pan. Turn gently to distribute and ensure everything is coated with the liquid.	
6	Sprinkle the remaining cheese on top.	
7	Bake until eggs are set, about 45 minutes. A knife inserted in the middle should come out clean at an internal temperature of 165°F	
8	For a double recipe, use a 9 x 13 in pan. Leftovers freeze and reheat well.	

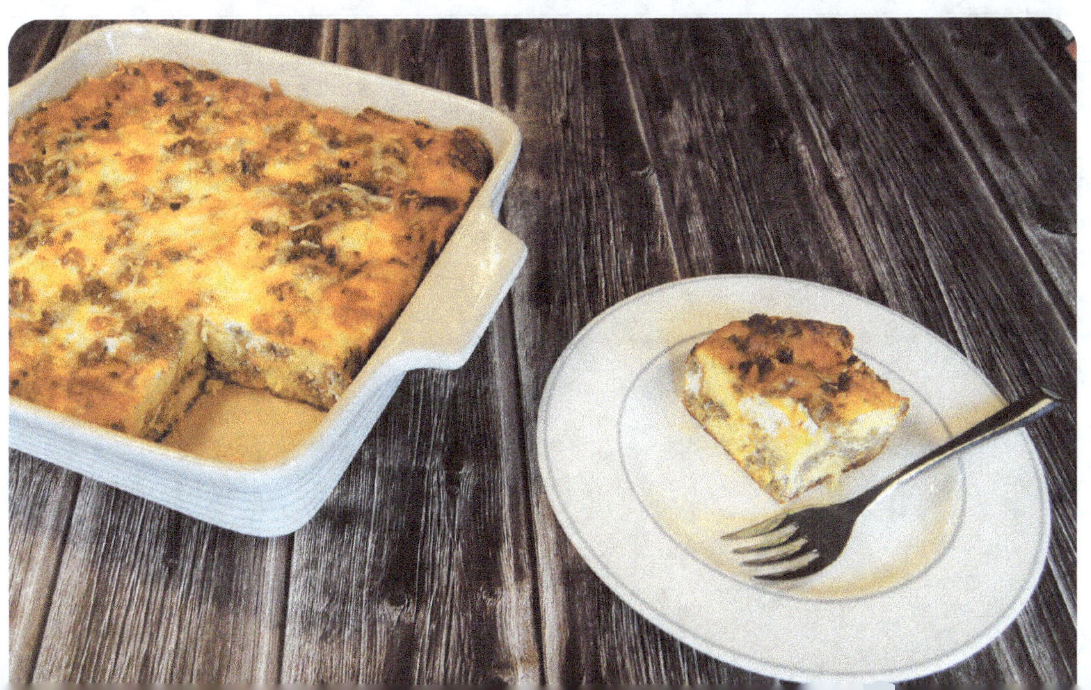

PROTEIN OTHER	**Spinach Mushroom Bake**[V] **Makes 12 servings**	**Breakfast**
INGREDIENTS		**SUBSTITUTE**
12	Eggs, large or XL	
16 oz	Cottage cheese	Ricotta cheese
16 oz	Shredded cheese, cheddar or blend	
8 Tbsp	Butter	
½ C	Corn starch	Tapioca flour or rice flour
10 oz	Chopped spinach, cooked and drained	
8 oz	Mushrooms, sliced	Fresh, frozen or canned
1	Onion, medium, diced	
1¼ tsp	Baking powder	
½ tsp	Salt	
½ tsp	Black pepper	
STEPS		
1	Preheat oven to 350°F. Prepare 9 x 13 inch pan by coating interior with oil.	
2	Sauté onion and mushrooms in butter until onion is soft. Add spinach and set aside to cool slightly.	
3	In a large bowl, whisk eggs then add cottage cheese, ¾ of the grated cheese, corn starch, baking powder, salt and pepper. Mix well.	
4	Stir spinach, onion and mushrooms into the egg mixture.	
5	Pour into prepared baking pan. Pan will be full.	
6	Spread remaining grated cheese on top.	
7	Bake until eggs are set and knife inserted into the center comes out clean, 45-60 minutes.	
8	Popular vegetarian and gluten free option for brunch. Leftovers freeze and reheat well.	

GRAIN	**Swedish Pancakes**[V] **Makes ~ twelve 6" pancakes**	**Breakfast**
INGREDIENTS		**SUBSTITUTE**
4	Eggs, large or XL	
1 tsp	Vanilla extract	
¼ C	Sugar	
2 C	Milk	
1½ C	Flour (180 g)	
3 Tbsp	Butter, melted	
STEPS		
1	Whisk eggs, vanilla and sugar together.	
2	Add milk and mix well.	
3	Add flour and whisk until smooth.	
4	Pour in melted butter slowly while continuing to stir. Batter will be thin. At this point, the batter may be stored in the refrigerator overnight.	
5	Preheat sauté pan lightly coated with oil over medium heat. The pan is hot enough when a drop of water will "dance".	
6	Pour about ⅓ C batter into hot pan, turning the pan so that the batter covers the entire bottom surface.	
7	Cook until the pancake is set, then flip to cook an additional couple minutes.	
8	Serve with your favorite topping: fruit and whipped cream, syrup, lingonberries, orange butter, chocolate-hazelnut spread, or powdered sugar.	

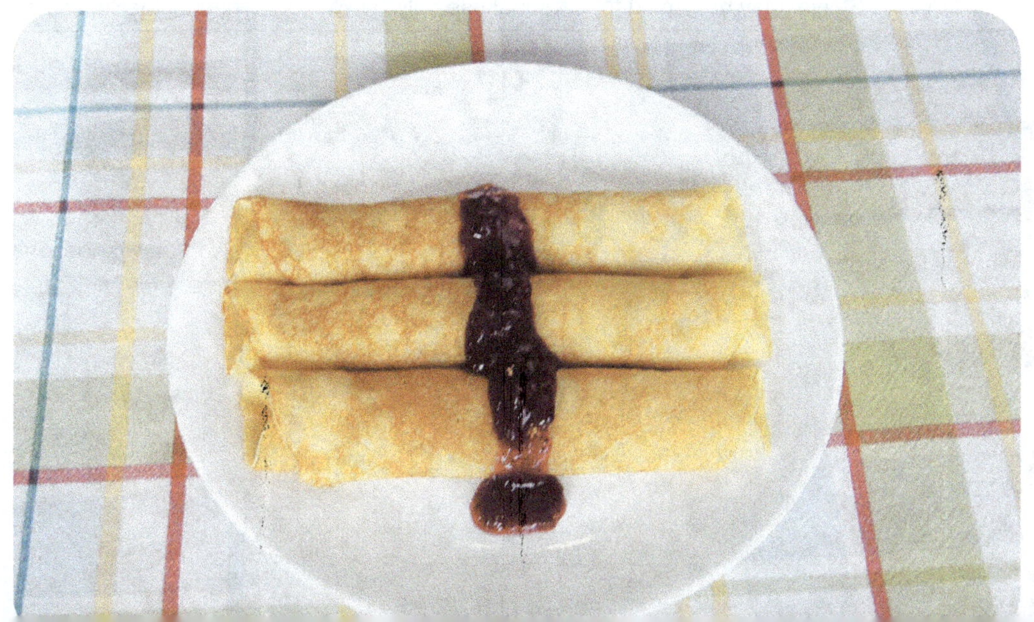

FRUIT	**Applesauce Oatmeal Crisp[V]** **Makes one 9" x 9" pan**	**Dessert**
INGREDIENTS		**SUBSTITUTE**
2½ C	Rolled oats (Old Fashioned or Quick)	
1 C	Brown sugar	White sugar
½ C	Butter, room temperature	Margarine (regular, not reduced fat)
24 oz	Applesauce, unsweetened (one jar)	Sweetened applesauce (reduce sugar by ⅓)
1 tsp	Cinnamon	Pumpkin pie spice
STEPS		
1	Preheat oven to 350°F.	
2	Mix oats, brown sugar and cinnamon together. Put ⅓ of the dry mixture in a 9" x 9" baking pan or 2½ quart baking dish.	
3	Pour applesauce over the dry oat mixture in the pan and mix.	
4	Add softened butter to the remaining dry oatmeal mixture and mix well. There should be no lumps of butter and the oats covered with butter. Spread over top of applesauce mixture.	
5	Bake for 45-60 minutes until top is crunchy and golden.	
6	Serve warm or cold, plain or garnished with whipped cream, ice cream or caramel sauce.	
OPTIONS		
A	**Additions**: Stir ⅓ C raisins, dried cranberries or cherries or chopped walnuts or pecans to the appleasauce mixture.	
B	**Extra Fruit**: Use a 46 oz jar of applesauce to increase the applesauce to topping ratio.	
C	**Any Fruit**: Replace the applesauce with Fast Fruit Filling (see recipe on page 67).	

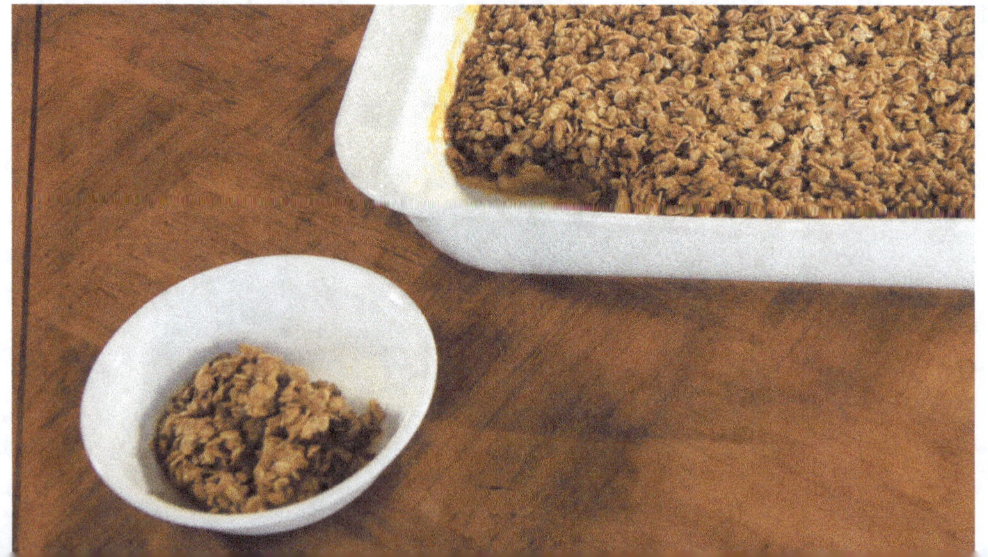

FRUIT	Bananas Foster[V] Serves 4	Dessert
INGREDIENTS		**SUBSTITUTE**
4	Bananas, peeled and sliced in half	
4 Tbsp	Butter	
½ C	Brown sugar, packed	
½ tsp	Cinnamon	
¼ C	Dark rum (optional)	Light rum or brandy
STEPS		
1	In a large skillet or sauté pan, melt butter and mix brown sugar and cinnamon in well.	
2	Over medium heat, add the banana slices to the bubbly butter/sugar mixture. Heat on each side for about 2 minutes. Bananas should start to caramelize.	
3	Pour rum over bananas and gently shake pan to mix.	
4	Optional Step: Flambe the rum upon addition by igniting it carefully with a long lighter. Flame should go out in just a few seconds.	
5	Serve warm over vanilla ice cream, pancakes, waffles, pound cake, or bread pudding.	

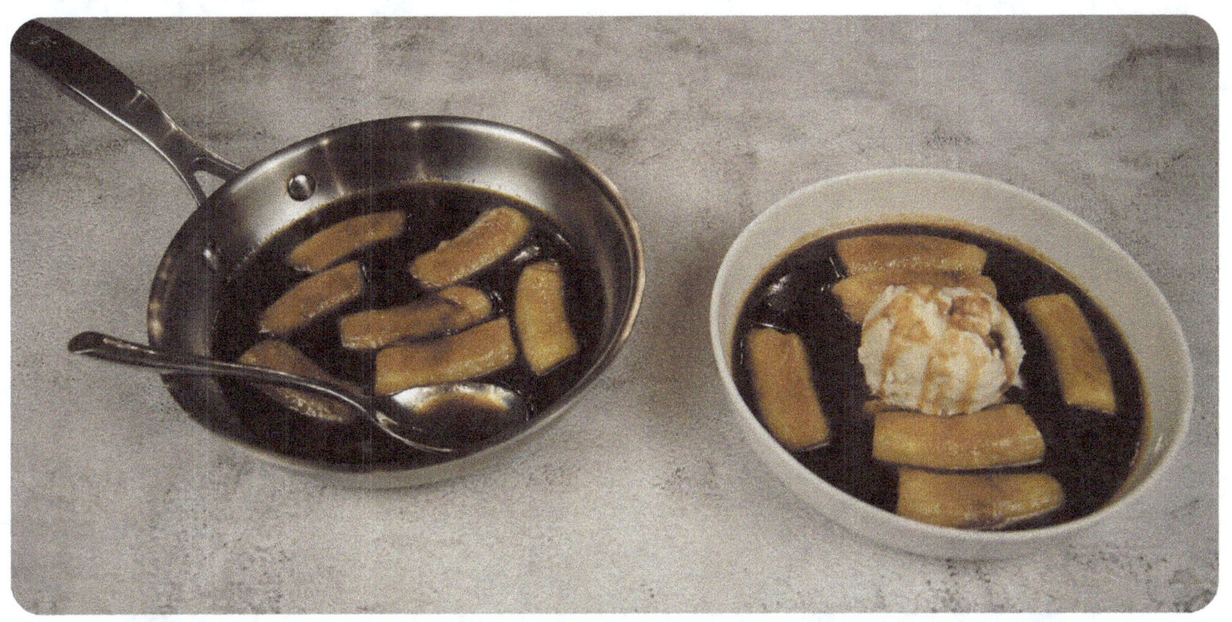

FRUIT	**Banana Pudding Parfait**[V] **Serves 4**	**Dessert**
INGREDIENTS		**SUBSTITUTE**
2 ½ C	Vanilla Milk Pudding - recipe on page 74	Any vanilla pudding
2	Bananas, sliced into coins	
30	Vanilla Wafers, coursley crushed	
4 Tbsp	Butter	
6 Tbsp	Brown sugar	
	Whipped cream for garnish	
STEPS		
1	Prepare vanilla pudding and set in fridge to cool.	
2	Melt butter in a sauté pan then add the brown sugar. Mix and heat to just bubbly but not carmelizing.	
3	Add cookie crumbs and continue to toast over medium heat, stirring constantly. Cook for 2-3 minutes then remove from heat.	
4	Prepare to assemble the parfait into four clear glasses (~12 oz) or one clear 1½ - 2 qt serving bowl.	
5	Reserve four rounded teaspoons of the cookie crumble for topping.	
6	Using half of the ingredients, make one layer of crumble - banana - pudding. Make a second layer using the rest of the ingredients.	
7	Garnish with whipped cream and 1 rounded teaspoon of crumble on top of each parfait.	

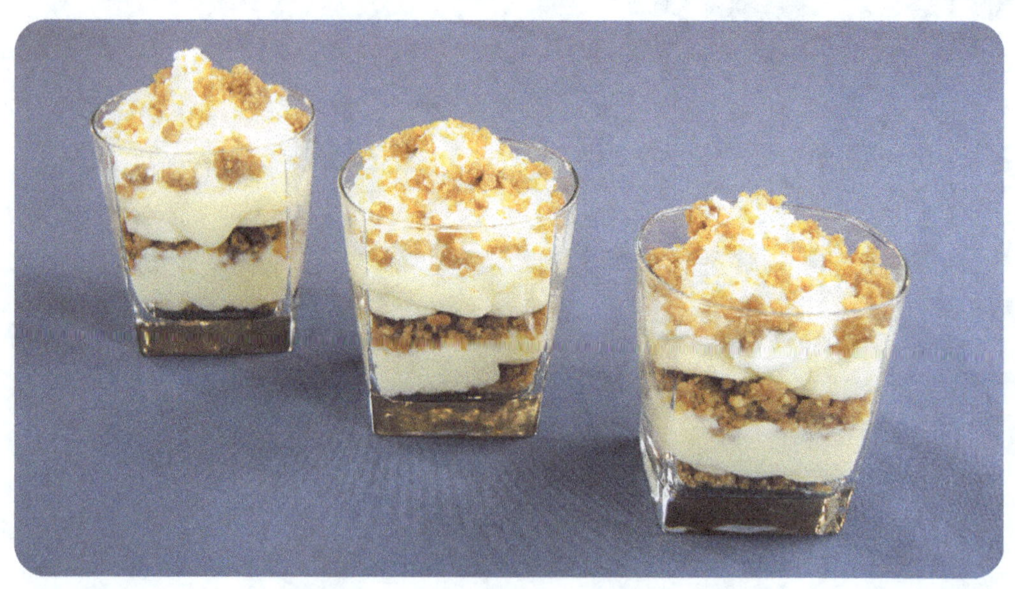

FRUIT	Brandied Peaches[V] Makes about 5 cups	Dessert
INGREDIENTS		**SUBSTITUTE**
4	Ripe peaches, medium to large	
1¾ C	White granulated sugar	
1½ C	Water	
2 tsp	Ground cloves	
½ C	Brandy	
STEPS		
1	Have clean glass jars with lids ready – mason jars or any heavy glass jars are fine.	
2	Clean the peaches well and cut into cubes or slices. They do not need to be peeled. Put peach pieces into glass jar(s), filling only ½ to ¾ full.	
3	In a sauce pan, heat water and sugar to boiling. It should thicken slightly, making a syrup that will coat the back of a spoon.	
4	Remove syrup from heat and stir in the ground cloves. Next stir in the brandy and mix well.	
5	When syrup is still warm, pour over the peaches. Cool before sealing the jars.	
6	Allow to set for at least 12 hours before serving. Store in the refrigerator for up to a week.	
7	Serve over vanilla ice cream, pancakes or french toast.	

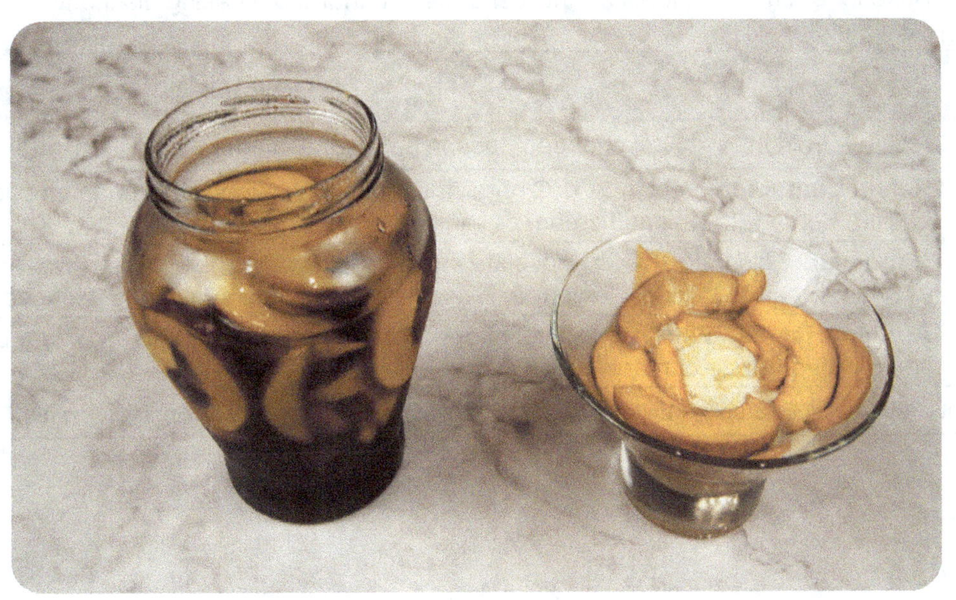

GRAIN	**Bread Pudding**[V] **Makes 8-12 servings**	**Dessert**
INGREDIENTS		**SUBSTITUTE**
12 oz	French bread, cut into 1 inch cubes	Any bread but stale and crusty is better
3 C	Milk	Half cream + half water
3	Eggs, large or XL	
½ - 1 C	Sugar	Brown sugar (affects appearance)
2 tsp	Vanilla extract	
½ tsp	Cinnamon	
¼ tsp	Nutmeg	
1-2 Tbsp	Butter, melted	

STEPS	
1	Preheat oven to 350°F.
2	In a large bowl, mix bread cubes and milk and allow to stand until milk is mostly absorbed.
3	In a second bowl, beat eggs, sugar and spices together.
4	Pour egg mixture over the bread and milk, then gently fold together. Ensure that the bread is well coated.
5	Prepare a 9 x 13 baking pan, casserole dish or individual baking dishes by coating interior with oil. Scoop mixture into pan. Drizzle with melted butter.
6	Bake for about 60 minutes or until center is set. Individual baking dishes will take closer to 50 minutes.

OPTIONS	
A	**Praline**: Fold in ½ -1 C of chopped pecans before baking then top with a caramel sauce.
B	**Raisin Cinnamon**: Fold in ½ -1 C of raisins and sprinkle top with cinnamon sugar before baking. Serve with whipped cream or vanilla ice cream.
C	**Chocolate**: Fold in ½ -1 C of chocolate chips or chocolate chunks (semi-sweet or dark chocolate) before baking. Serve with a drizzle of chocolate sauce and whipped cream.
D	**Autumn Harvest**: Fold in ½ -1 C of chopped dried apricots or cherries before baking then serve with a drizzle of maple syrup.

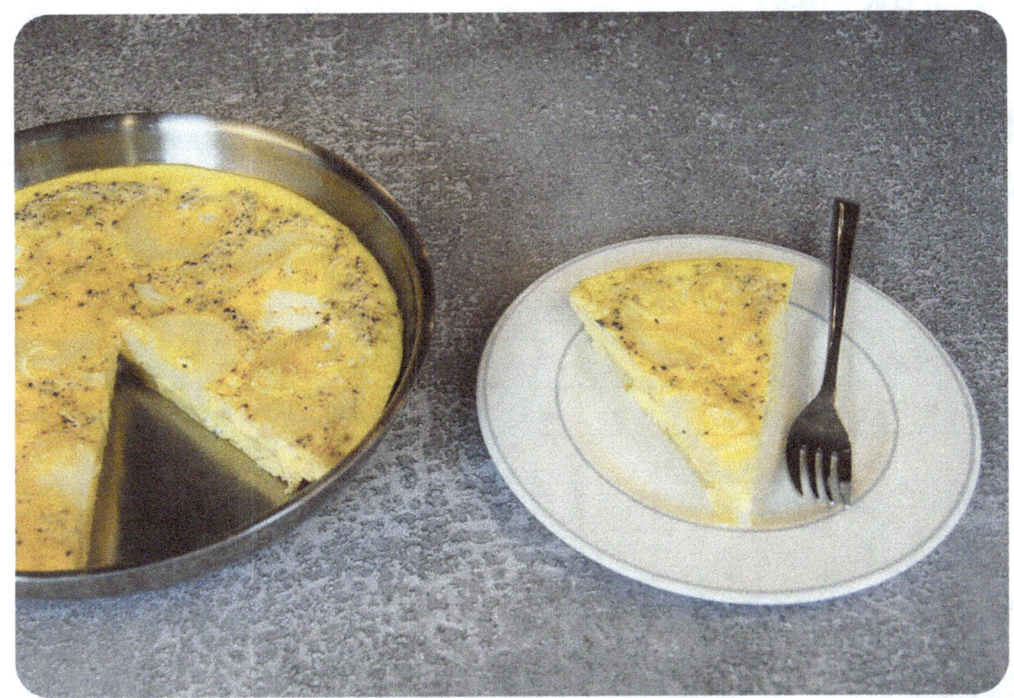

Potato Frittata

Recipe on page 56

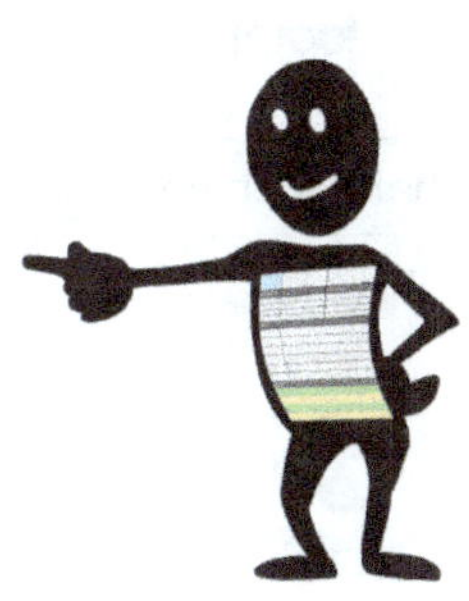

Bread Pudding

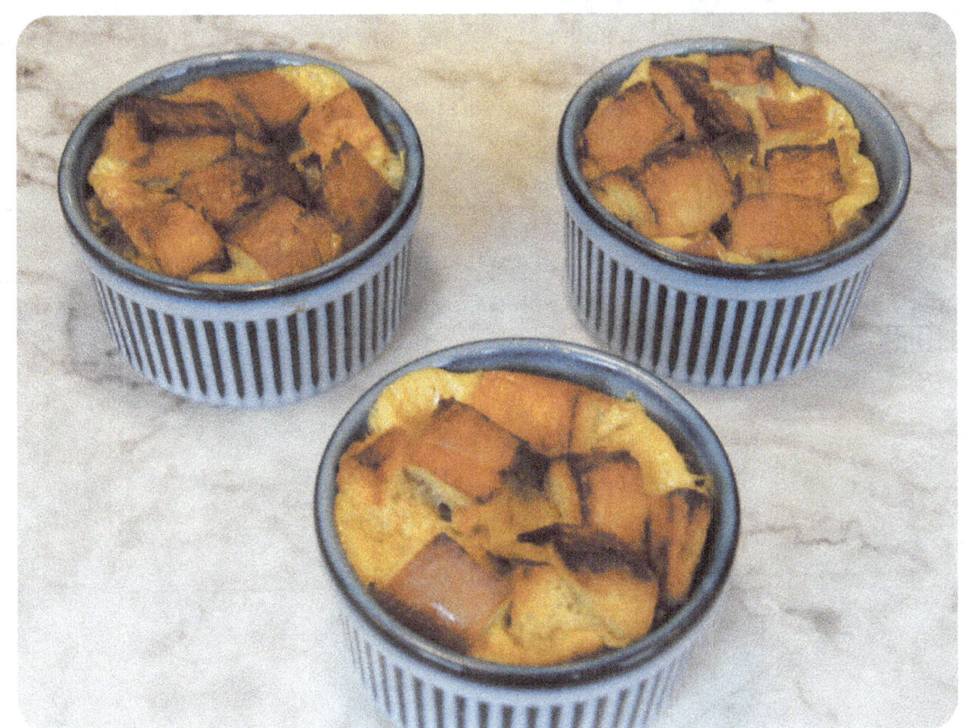

GRAIN	Brownies[V] Makes one 8” x 8” pan	Dessert
INGREDIENTS		**SUBSTITUTE**
½ C	Butter, room temperature	Margarine or coconut oil
1 C	Sugar	½ C white sugar + ½ C brown sugar
2	Eggs, large or XL	
1 tsp	Vanilla extract	
½ C	Baking cocoa, unsweetened	Dark chocolate baking cocoa
½ C	Flour, all purpose (60 g)	Self rising flour (omit baking powder and salt)
1 tsp	Baking powder	
½ tsp	Salt	
½ C	Chocolate chips (optional)	Any flavor baking chips, M&Ms, crushed candy canes
½ C	Chopped nuts (optional)	
STEPS		
1	Preheat oven to 350°F. Prepare a 8” x 8” pan by coating with cooking spray. Use a 9’ x 13” pan for a double recipe.	
2	In a bowl, beat the sugar and butter together then add eggs and vanilla. Beat with a whisk or mixer until fully incorporated.	
3	Stir cocoa, flour, baking powder and salt together in a small bowl then pour into the egg mixture and mix until smooth.	
4	Fold optional chocolate chips and/or nuts into batter, if using.	
5	Spread batter in pan and bake for 20-25 minutes. Brownies are done when a toothpick inserted in the middle comes out clean. Cool before cutting.	

GRAIN	Butter Berry Cobbler[V] Makes 8 - 12 servings	Dessert
INGREDIENTS		**SUBSTITUTE**
8 Tbsp	Butter	Margarine
2 C	Flour, all purpose (240 g)	Up to ⅓ whole wheat
1 Tbsp	Baking powder	
2 C	Sugar (white or brown)	Reduce by ½ C for a less sweet result
2 C	Milk	
¼ tsp	Salt	
16 oz	Any Berries, fresh or frozen (3-4 C)	Canned or frozen peaches
STEPS		
1	Preheat oven to 350°F.	
2	Thaw fruit if using frozen.	
3	Put butter in 9 x 13 inch pan then place in oven to melt butter and heat pan.	
4	In a bowl, mix the flour, salt, baking powder and sugar.	
5	Stir in the milk and mix. It is OK to leave slightly lumpy.	
6	Remove hot pan from oven with melted butter. Pour the batter mixture into pan – do not stir.	
7	Drop fruit into batter, evenly distributing over the entire surface. Any residual fruit juice may be drizzled in, avoiding the center.	
8	Bake for 50-60 minutes until golden brown and center is firm.	
9	Serve warm or cool. Great with vanilla ice cream.	

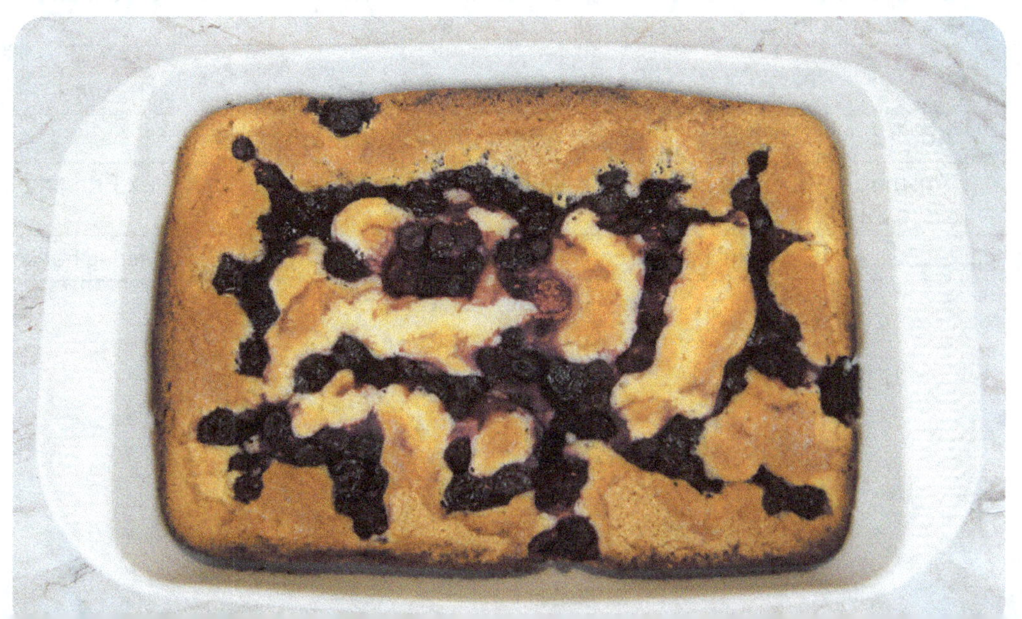

GRAIN	Chocolate Applesauce Cake[V] Makes one 9" x 9" cake	Dessert
INGREDIENTS		**SUBSTITUTE**
2 C	All purpose flour (240 g)	Substitute up to one half whole wheat flour.
1-1½ C	Sugar	
3 Tbsp	Cocoa powder	
1 Tbsp	Baking soda	
1 tsp	Cinnamon	
½ tsp	Nutmeg	
½ tsp	Cloves	
¼ tsp	Salt	
1 Tbsp	Corn starch	
½ C	Vegetable oil	Melted butter
2 C	Applesauce, unsweetened	Sweetened applesauce (use ½ C less sugar)
STEPS		
1	Preheat oven to 325°F.	
2	Prepare pan (either bundt pan or 9 x 9 baking pan) by coating with oil then dusting with flour.	
3	Place all dry ingredients in bowl and mix well.	
4	Warm applesauce and oil together in oven or microwave to about 110°F.	
5	Add applesauce and oil to the dry ingredients and mix thoroughly.	
6	Pour batter into prepared baking pan.	
7	Bake for one hour. Check for doneness after 45 minutes. A knife or toothpick inserted in the middle should come out clean when cake is done.	
OPTIONS		
A	**Additions**: Add ½ C of chopped nuts or raisins or dried cranberries.	
B	**Toppings**: Whipped cream or fresh berries or lemon curd or Fast Flex Frosting shown on page 221.	

Photo on page 72

PROTEIN OTHER	**Egg Custard**[V] **Makes 6-8 cups**	**Dessert**
INGREDIENTS		**SUBSTITUTE**
3 C	Milk	Commercially prepared eggnog (omit sugar)
½ C	Sugar	
4	Eggs, large or XL	
1	Egg white	
1 tsp	Vanilla extract	
STEPS		
1	Preheat oven to 325°F.	
2	Mix all ingredients and beat well. May be done with a blender, mixer or whisk.	
3	Place 6-8 custard cups into a shallow baking pan. Fill each cup with 4-5½ oz of the mixture.	
4	Pour about 1 inch of hot water into the baking pan so that the cups are surrounded by water.	
5	Carefully set pan with the water and cups into the oven. Bake for 45-60 minutes, until the custard has just set. A knife inserted into the custard will come out clean.	
6	Remove from oven and allow to cool. Cover and chill before serving.	
7	Serve plain or with a sprinkle of nutmeg, cinnamon sugar, caramel sauce, fruit preserves or fresh berries.	

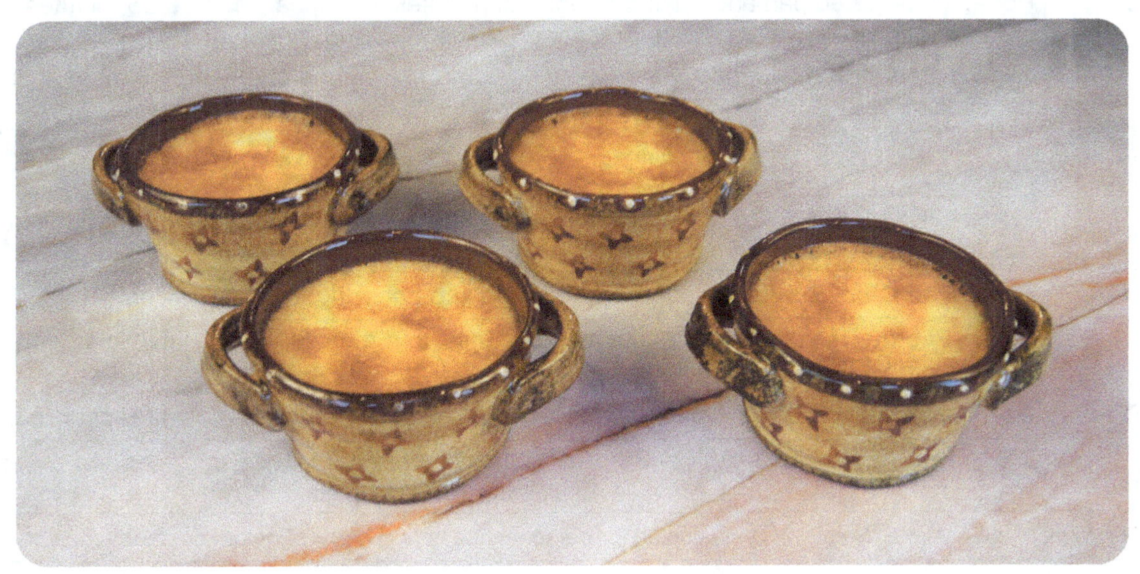

GRAIN	**Essential Cake**[V] **Makes one 8" - 9" cake**	**Dessert**
INGREDIENTS		**SUBSTITUTE**
8 Tbsp	Butter, softened	Margarine
¾ C	White sugar	Brown sugar
2	Large or XL eggs, room temperature	
1½ tsp	Vanilla extract	Almond or other flavor extract
1½ C	All Purpose Flour or Cake Flour (180 g)	1 C rice flour + ½ C tapicoa flour (GF)
1½ tsp	Baking powder	
½ tsp	Salt	
¾ C	Milk	Buttermilk
STEPS		
1	Preheat oven to 350°F.	
2	Prepare pan by coating with oil (or cooking spray) and then dusting with flour. May use 8-9 inch square or round pan, loaf pan or 12 cupcake pan.	
3	In a large bowl, beat butter and sugar until it is well combined, light and fluffy.	
4	Add eggs to the bowl and beat well. Add vanilla extact and beat.	
5	Measure flour (weighing is best), baking powder and salt into a bowl and stir to mix.	
6	Add half of the flour and half of the milk to the butter/egg bowl then beat to incorporate. Add remaining flour and milk and beat until batter is smooth, about two minutes.	
7	Pour into prepared pan and bake for about 20 minutes for cupcakes or 30-35 minutes for a pan. Cake is done when a toothpick inserted in the middle comes out clean.	
8	Allow to cool. May be topped with frosting, ice cream, whipped cream, fruit compote, caramel or chocolate sauce.	
OPTIONS		
A	**Confetti Cake**: Stir ¼ C colorful sprinkles into batter right before baking. Frost with vanilla frosting and decorate with more sprinkles.	
B	**Chocolate Chip**: Stir ½ C mini chocolate chips into batter right before baking.	
C	**Maple Pecan**: Use maple extract instead of vanilla and then stir in ½ C finely chopped pecans into batter right before baking.	
D	**Berry**: Wash & dry one cup of blueberries or raspberries & fold into the batter prior to baking.	
E	**Cinnamon Coffee Cake**: Mix ½ C brown sugar, 2 tsp cinnamon, 2 Tbsp flour and 3 Tbsp melted butter together, then sprinkle over batter prior to baking.	

	Fast Flex Frosting[V] **Makes ~ 3 cups**	**Dessert**
INGREDIENTS		**SUBSTITUTE**
2-3	Sticks butter - softened (unsalted preferred)	Margarine, Crisco
0-1	Package (8 oz) cream cheese - softened	
4 C	Powdered sugar	Use 1¼ C brown or white granulated sugar (affects texture)
1½ tsp	Vanilla extract	Other extract - lemon, almond
STEPS		
1	Use 3 sticks of butter or 2 sticks of butter plus one package cream cheese.	
2	Beat butter and cream cheese (if using) in bowl with mixer until fluffy.	
3	Add vanilla extract.	
4	Add powdered sugar in four increments, beating well between additions. Frosting should be firm yet spreadable.	
5	Adjust consistency: Add sugar in 1 Tbsp increments to thicken or milk by 1 tsp increments to thin.	
6	Yields about 3 cups of frosting. Enough for 24 cupcakes (2 Tbsp each) or one 9" x 13" sheet cake.	
OPTIONS		
A	**Spread**: Can be made with white granulated sugar or brown sugar (reduce volume). However, the texture will be softer, and a bit grainy. Tastes ok in a pinch but not workable for decorating.	
B	**Lemon**: Use 2 tsp lemon extract instead of vanilla, and for extra flavor, add 1 Tbsp lemon zest.	
C	**Chocolate**: Add ½ C melted chocolate chips to the butter/cream cheese mixture in step 3. Add vanilla and sugar as usual.	
D	**Almond**: Use 2 tsp almond extract in place of vanilla. Use almond slices as decoration.	

Photos of Essential Cake and Fast Flex Frosting on page 72

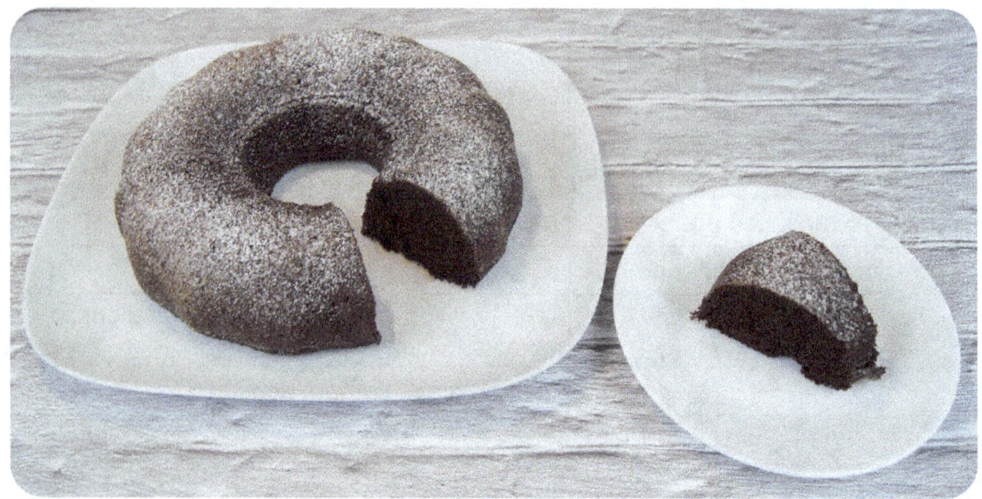

Chocolate Applesauce Cake

Recipe on page 69

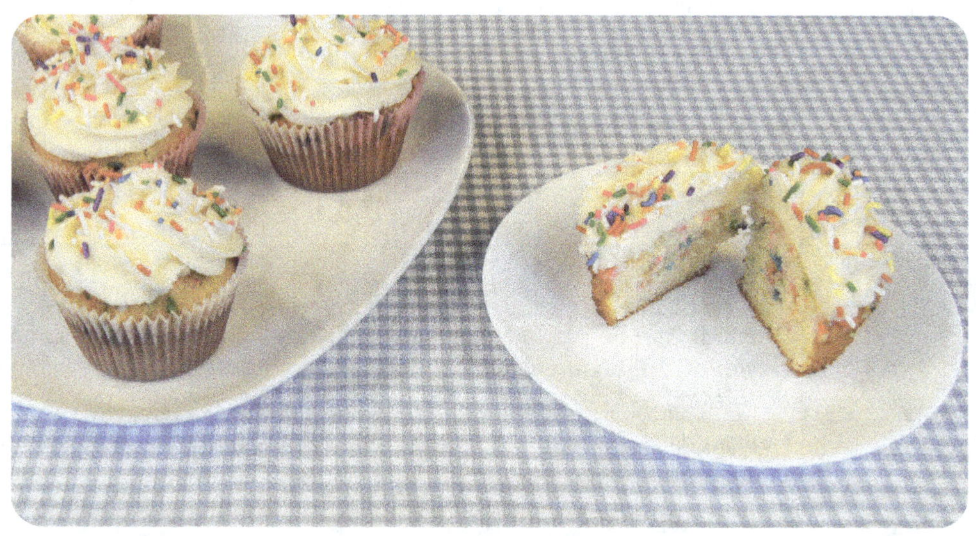

Essential Cake & Fast Flex Frosting - Recipes on pages 70 & 71

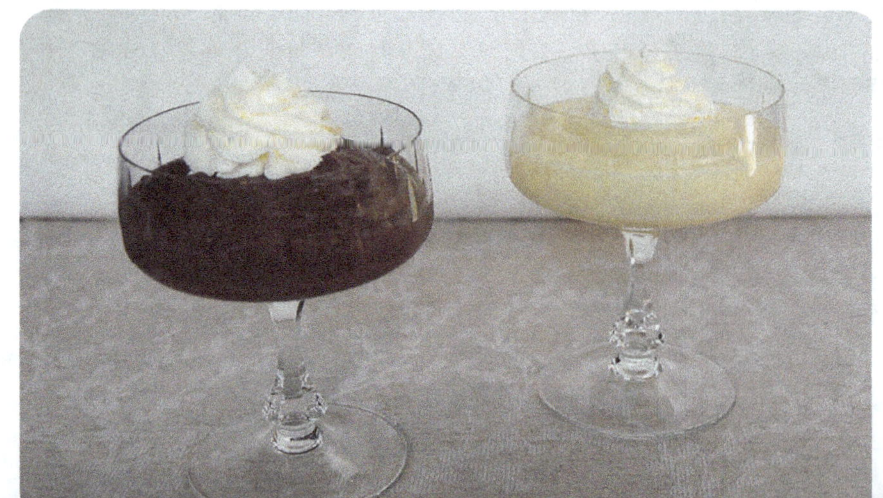

Milk Pudding

Vanilla & Chocolate

Recipe on page 74

FRUIT	Fast Fruit Filling[V] Makes 1¾ cups	Dessert
INGREDIENTS		**SUBSTITUTE**
1	Bag (16 oz) frozen berries	Any non-citrus frozen, fresh (A) or canned fruit (B)
½ C	Sugar	Any natural or artificial sweetener. If using liquid, add 1 tsp corn starch per ½ C liquid.
2 Tbsp	Corn starch	Rice flour
1 tsp	Lemon juice	Any juice or OJ concentrate
STEPS		
1	In a heat-proof glass bowl or measuring cup, microwave fruit for 3 minutes on high until thawed but still cold.	
2	Stir sugar, lemon juice and corn starch into fruit and mix well.	
3	Microwave on high for four minutes then stir.	
4	Microwave on high for another four minutes. Should be steamy and look glossy.	
5	If it is not yet steamy and glossy, continue heating in microwave in one minute increments until it is.	
6	Serve hot or cold. Makes about 1¾ Cups.	
7	Use as a topping for ice cream, pancakes, french toast, or cheesecake. Layer in a parfait or to fill a pie shell or tart shell. Use as a fruity complement to roast poultry or pork.	
OPTIONS		
A	**Fresh Fruit**: Skip the initial thawing step and add 2-5 minutes to the microwave time until fruit is cooked and thickened.	
B	**Canned Fruit**: Skip the initial thawing step, reduce sugar if fruit is sweetened, and add 1 Tbsp more cornstarch.	
C	**Spices**: Add 1 tsp cinnamon, nutmeg, ginger or other spices to complement fruit.	
D	**Liquor**: For a sophistiacted flavor, add 2 Tbsp liquor and an additional 1 tsp cornstarch in step 2. Grand Marnier, brandy, Amaretto and Chambord are suggestions.	

Photo on page 72

PROTEIN OTHER	**Milk Pudding^{V}** **Makes about 2½ cups**	**Dessert**
INGREDIENTS		**SUBSTITUTE**
2 C	Milk	1 C cream + 1 C water, almond or oat milk
½ C	Sugar	
2 Tbsp	Corn starch	
2	Eggs, large or XL	
1 tsp	Vanilla extract	
STEPS		
1	In a medium sauce pan, mix cold milk, corn starch and sugar well. Bring mixture to almost a boil over medium heat stirring constantly. It will start to thicken. Remove from heat.	
2	In a small bowl, beat eggs.	
3	Temper the eggs by slowly adding a cup of hot milk mixture to the eggs, 1-2 tablespoons at a time while stirring briskly.	
4	Pour tempered egg mixture back into the warm milk mixture in the pan stirring constantly.	
5	Cook over low heat stirring continuously until pudding almost boils and it thickens. Pudding will thicken more as it cools.	
6	Remove from heat and stir in the vanilla extract. Cover when cool. Serve warm or cold.	
OPTIONS		
A	**Vanilla Pudding**: Recipe above. Serve plain or with whipped cream, berries, or in a parfait.	
B	**Chocolate Pudding**: Stir ⅔ C chocolate chips or small pieces of chocolate bar into hot pudding. Stir to mix melted chocolate into pudding.	
C	**Maple Brown Sugar Pudding**: Use brown sugar instead of white sugar and stir in 1 tsp of maple extract along with the vanilla extract.	
D	**Fruity Parfait**: Layer pudding with fresh fruit, canned fruit, or jam, and granola or crushed cookies.	

Why make pudding from scratch?

- **It is super easy and you already have all the ingredients.**
- **This recipe has about 8 g of protein per serving.**
- **It costs about half vs making pudding from a mix.**
- **There are no artificial ingredients.**

Photo on page 72

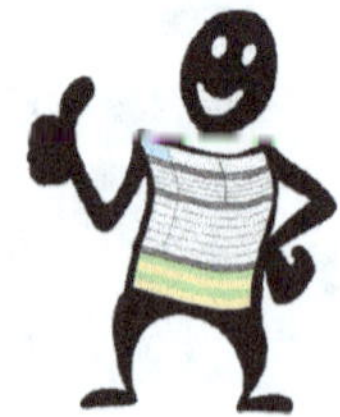

GRAIN	**Pantry Cake[V]** **Makes one 8” x 8” cake**	**Dessert**
INGREDIENTS		**SUBSTITUTE**
1½ C	Flour, all purpose (180 g)	
5 Tbsp	Cocoa powder	
¾ C	White sugar	
1 tsp	Baking powder	
½ tsp	Salt	
1 C	Coffee, cold	Water
1 tsp	Vanilla extract	
2 tsp	Vinegar, white	Apple cider vinegar
⅓ C	Canola oil	Coconut oil, melted butter
STEPS		
1	Preheat oven to 350°F. Prepare a 8” x 8” pan by coating with cooking spray.	
2	Whisk dry ingredients in a bowl to combine well.	
3	Add liquid ingredients to dry and mix well with a whisk or large fork until there are no lumps.	
4	Pour into prepared pan.	
5	Bake for 25-30 minutes or until a toothpick comes out clean. Allow to cool before frosting or cutting.	
6	Serve topped with a sprinkle of powdered sugar, whipped cream or any frosting.	

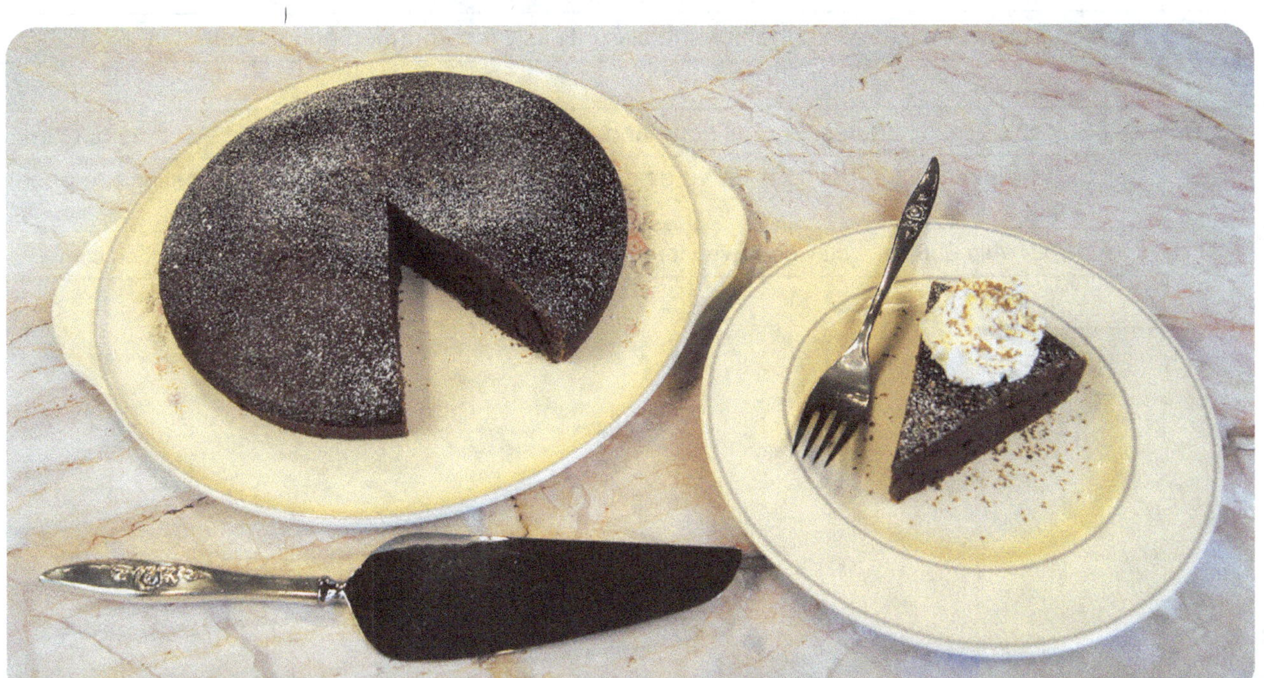

GRAIN	Pumpkin Muffins[V] Makes 24 muffins	Dessert
INGREDIENTS		**SUBSTITUTE**
2 C + 1½ Tbsp	Flour, all purpose (251 g)	1½ C rice flour + ⅔ C tapioca flour or corn starch
1½ tsp	Baking powder	
½ tsp	Baking soda	
1 tsp	Salt	
1½ tsp	Ginger	
1 tsp	Cinnamon	
½ tsp	Cloves, ground	
½ tsp	Nutmeg	
¾ C	Sugar, white	
¾ C	Sugar, brown	
1 C	Butter, melted	Light vegetable oil
4	Eggs, large or XL	
1	Pumpkin puree, 15 oz can	

STEPS	
1	Preheat oven to 350°F. Prepare muffin pans by coating with cooking spray or using paper liners.
2	In a large bowl, mix the flour, baking powder, baking soda and spices together.
3	In a second bowl, mix the sugars, butter, eggs and pumpkin puree together.
4	Pour the wet mixture into the dry and stir until fully incorporated and smooth.
5	Pour batter info the muffin pans.
6	Bake for 20-25 minutes, or until done and a toothpick inserted in the middle comes out clean.
7	Serve plain or add frosting to serve as cupcakes (vanilla or cream cheese frosting are good choices).

GRAIN	**Rice Pudding[V]** **Makes ~ 5 cups**	**Dessert**
INGREDIENTS		**SUBSTITUTE**
3 C	Cooked rice (white or brown)	Quinoa or wild rice
2 C	Milk	Almond or oat milk or half cream and half water.
½-1 C	Sugar	
2	Eggs, large or XL	
1 tsp	Vanilla extract	
STEPS		
1	In a medium suace pan, bring rice, milk and sugar almost to a boil, stirring constantly.	
2	Reduce heat and simmer for 15 minutes, stirring often.	
3	In a small bowl, beat eggs.	
4	Temper the eggs by adding a cup of hot milk/rice mixture to the eggs, 1-2 tablespoons at a time while stirring well.	
5	Pour tempered egg mixture back into warm pan and mix well.	
6	Cook over low heat for about 5 minutes stirring continuously.	
7	Remove from heat and stir in the vanilla extract. Allow to cool then cover. Serve warm or cold, sprinkled with nutmeg or cinnamon sugar.	
OPTIONS		
A	**Chocloate Rice Pudding**: Stir ½ C chocolate chips or pieces of chocolate bar into hot pudding.	
B	**Additions**: Stir in ⅓ C raisins or other dried fruit.	

PROTEIN OTHER	Ricotta Cheesecake[V] Makes one 9" cake	Dessert
INGREDIENTS		**SUBSTITUTE**
32 oz	Ricotta cheese, well drained	
1½ C	Powdered sugar	½ C sugar
4	Eggs, large or XL	
2 Tbsp	Corn starch	
1 tsp	Almond extract	1 Tbsp lemon or orange zest, 1 Tbsp Amaretto or Grand Mariner
STEPS		
1	Preheat oven to 350°F.	
2	Prepare 9 inch springform pan by either coating it with butter and then flour, or lining it with parchment paper.	
3	In a bowl, beat the ricotta cheese and sugar until smooth.	
4	Add the eggs, corn starch and extract and beat gently until fully combined.	
5	Pour batter into the prepared pan.	
6	Bake about 60 minutes or until the center of the cake is just set. Cool fully before cutting. Serve plain or with a dusting of powdered sugar, whipped cream and berries.	

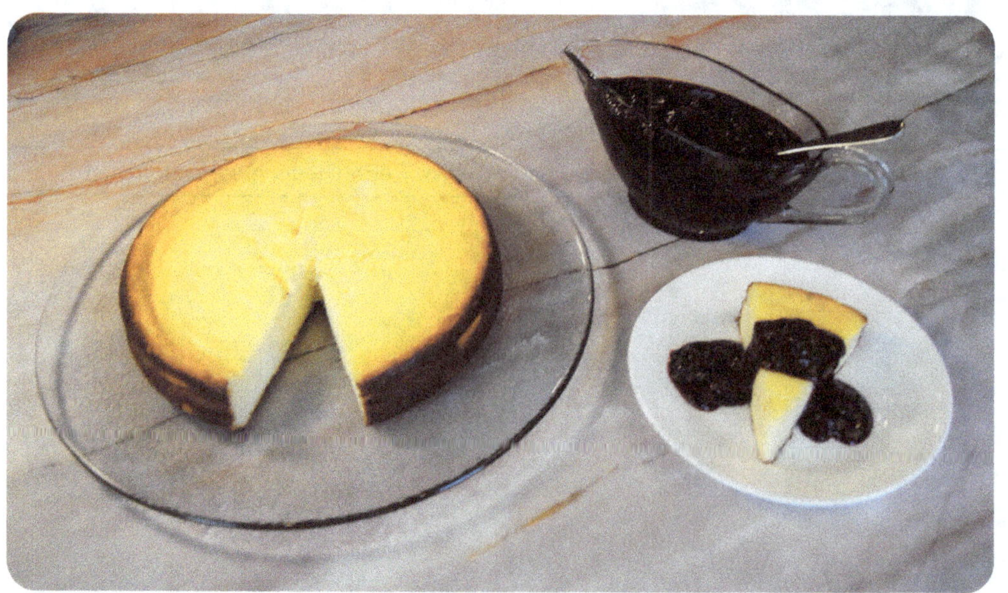

Shown with

Fast Fruit Filling

Recipe on page 67

GRAIN	Russian Tea Cakes[V] Makes ~ 24	Dessert
INGREDIENTS		**SUBSTITUTE**
1 C	Butter, room temperature	
½ C	Confectioners sugar (plus more for coating)	
1 tsp	Vanilla extract	
2½ C	All purpose flour (300 g)	2¾ C cake flour or substitute up to one fourth whole wheat flour
¼ tsp	Salt	
¾ C	Finely chopped walnuts or pecans	Almond meal (nuts are not optional)
STEPS		
1	Preheat oven to 400°F. Line cookie sheet with parchment paper if desired.	
2	In a large mixing bowl, cream butter, sugar and vanilla with mixer until smooth. A hand whisk may be used with good vigor.	
3	Add salt and flour. If you have a scale, you can weigh the flour directly into the bowl. Mix well.	
4	Add nuts and mix well. Dough should come together but be crumbly.	
5	Scoop rounded tablespoons of dough and roll into ~1" balls. Place on ungreased cookie sheet.	
6	Bake for 10-16 minutes, until set but not brown.	
7	Roll in confectioners sugar while warm and then again when cool. Store tightly covered.	

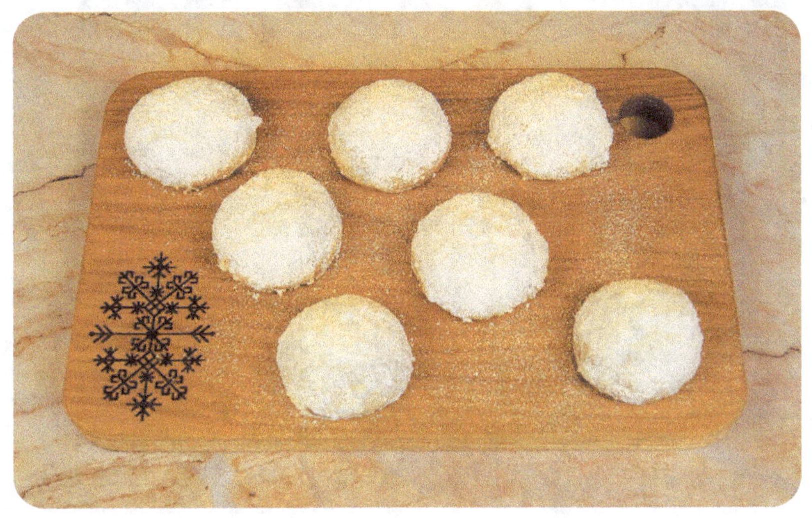

FRUIT	**Spiced Poached Fruit**[V] **Makes 4-6 servings**	**Dessert**
INGREDIENTS		**SUBSTITUTE**
1½ C	White wine	
½ C	Water	
¾ C	White sugar	Brown sugar
1 Tbsp	Ginger paste or minced candied ginger	Cinnamon
3 C	Fresh fruit - apple, peach, or pineapple	
STEPS		
1	In a sauce pan boil wine, water and sugar until it reduces slightly and starts to thicken, about 15 minutes.	
2	Remove from heat and stir in the ginger or other spice.	
3	Cut the fruit into slices or chunks and place in a heat resistant covered dish.	
4	Pour hot liquid over fruit, cover and allow to cool to room temperature. Refrigerate for an additional 1-24 hours.	
5	Served chilled fruit and syrup over ice cream or sorbet.	

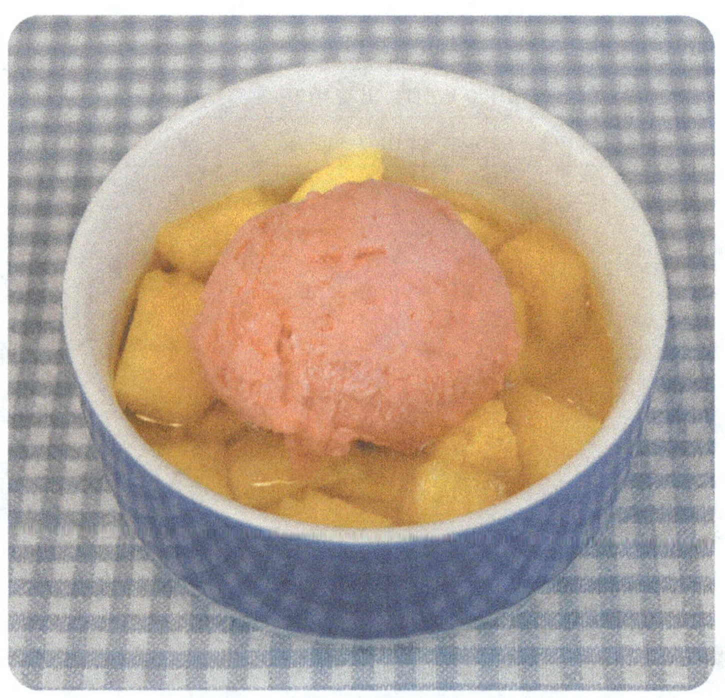

"Anything worth cooking generally starts with sautéed onion and garlic."

- Bette C. Martinoff

GRAIN	5-Minute Flatbread[V] Serves 2	Main
INGREDIENTS		**SUBSTITUTE**
2	Naan, fresh or frozen	Any flat bread, wrap or wheat tortilla
½ C	Marinara sauce or pizza sauce	See Instant Marinara Sauce recipe page 143
2 oz	Pepperoni	Hard salami
6 oz	Mozzarella, grated	
STEPS		
1	Preheat oven to 400°F and line a baking sheet with parchment paper.	
2	Spread sauce over the top of the bread then add the toppings and cheese.	
3	Bake for 5-8 minutes, or until cheese is melted and bubbly.	
OPTIONS		
A	**BBQ**: Replace marinara suace with BBQ sauce, use cooked diced chicken or pork instead of pepperoni, and cheddar cheese instead of mozzarella. Sliced red onion is nice.	
B	**Veggie**: Replace pepperoni with thinly sliced veggies such as mushrooms, onion, peppers, spinach	
C	**Caprese**: Replace marinara with pesto and top with slices of fresh tomato and fresh mozzarella.	

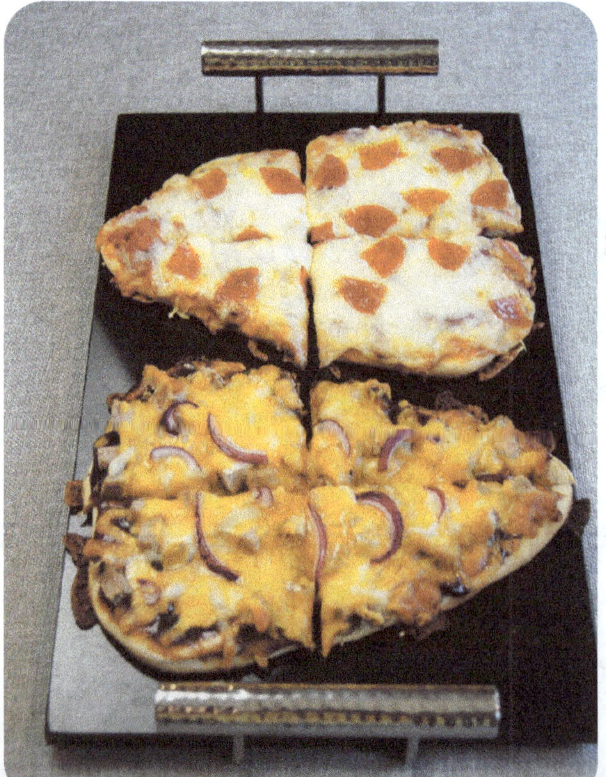

Marinara Pepperoni

Option A - BBQ

PROTEIN MEAT	**Apricot Glazed Pork Tenderloin** **Serves 6-8**	**Main**
INGREDIENTS		**SUBSTITUTE**
2	Pork tenderloins, about 1 lb each	
1 tsp	Salt	
½ tsp	Black pepper, ground	
1	18 oz jar apricot preserves	Cherry preserves
1 tsp	Garlic, minced	
2 tsp	Dijon mustard	
1½ tsp	Herbs de Provence	Rosemary or thyme
4 Tbsp	Sherry or any red wine	White wine, broth, or juice
STEPS		
1	Preheat oven to 400°F. Grease a shallow 9 x 13 baking dish.	
2	Season pork with salt and pepper.	
3	Roast pork for 10 minutes.	
4	Combine all other ingredients in a small sauce pan, mix well, and bring to a boil..	
5	Spoon about ½ of the apricot mixture over the pork and return to the oven for an additional 20-30 minutes. Medium will be at an internal temp of 145°F and well at 165°F.	
6	Allow pork to rest for 5 minutes before slicing. Serve with the remaining apricot sauce on the side.	

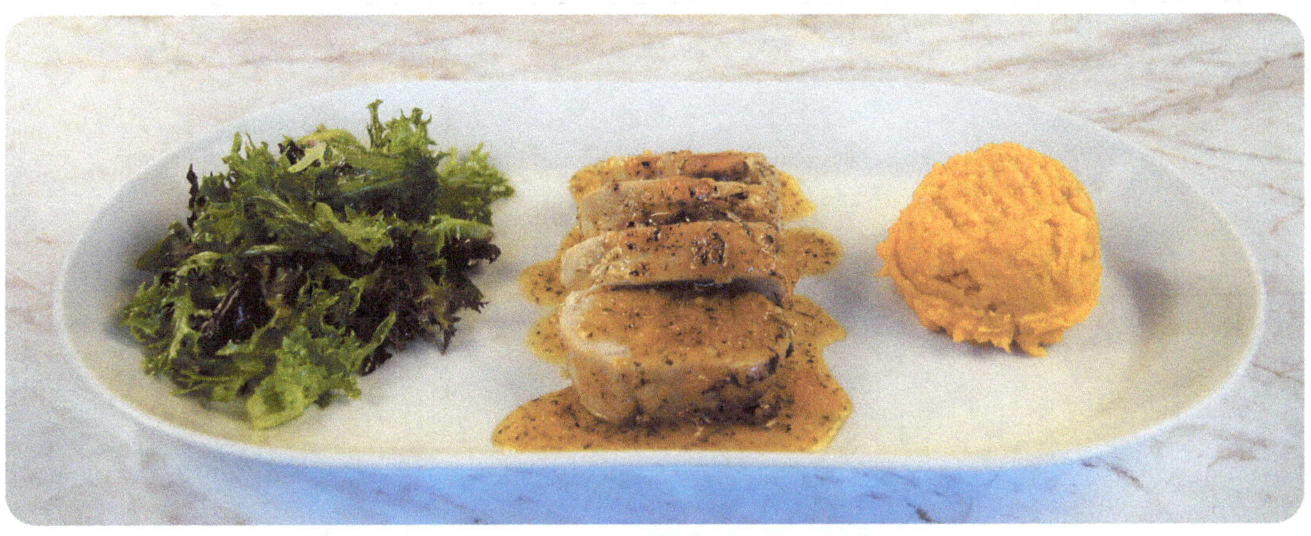

PROTEIN MEAT	Asian Glazed Anything[V] Serves 3-4	Main
INGREDIENTS		**SUBSTITUTE**
1 lb	Chicken breast	Firm tofu, steak, pork, shrimp
1 Tbsp	Canola oil	Peanut oil
4 Tbsp	Soy sauce	
3 Tbsp	Water	
2 Tbsp	Brown sugar	
2	Cloves garlic, minced	1 tsp jarred minced garlic
1 tsp	Sesame oil	
1 tsp	Chili sauce	½ tsp red pepper flakes
1 Tbsp	Corn starch	
¼ C	Green onions, sliced	
STEPS		
1	Cut the meat or tofu into 1/2 inch thick slices. Leave shrimp whole.	
2	In a large skillet, heat the oil to shimmering. Add meat and cook over medium high heat for three minutes per side. Should be nicely browned and almost completely cooked.	
3	Whisk together remaining ingredients except green onions in a small bowl. Corn starch should form a smooth slurry.	
4	Add sauce to the pan and continue to cook for about three minutes, stirring. Sauce should thicken.	
5	Serve with white rice and garnished with green onions.	

GRAIN	Baked Rice Casserole[V] Serves 6-8	Main
INGREDIENTS		**SUBSTITUTE**
4 C	Cooked rice, white or brown	Packaged cooked rice, microwaved
1 lb	Cooked chicken, diced or shredded	Two 12.5 oz cans of chicken meat, cooked turkey or roast pork
½	Onion, finely diced	2 Tbsp dehydrated onion
4 C	Broccoli or broccolini, cut into bite size pieces	12 oz bag of frozen broccoli florets
4 C	Milk	
4 Tbsp	Flour	
2 C	Cheddar cheese, grated (8 oz)	Co-Jack cheese
1 Tbsp	Mushroom seasoning	Complete seasoning or other seasoning blend.
2 tsp	Salt (omit if your seasoning has salt in it)	
1 C	Panko bread crumbs (optional)	Any bread or cracker crumbs
STEPS		
1	Preheat oven to 350°F. Prepare a 9" x 13" pan or 2-3 qt baking dish by coating with cooking spray.	
2	In a cup or bowl, mix the flour and milk together until a smooth, lump free slurry is achieved.	
3	In a large stock pot, pour the milk and flour slurry together with the remaining milk and cook over medium heat until the mixture starts to thicken. Stir in the seasoning and salt.	
4	Add the rice, chicken, onion, broccoli and half of the cheese to the milk mixture and stir to mix.	
5	Pour rice mixture into the baking dish and top with remaining cheese and bread crumbs (if using)	
6	Bake for 45 minutes or until bubbly and golden on top.	
OPTIONS		
A	**Chicken Pot Pie Rice**: Replace broccoli with peas and carrots (thawed, if frozen) and replace mushroom seasoning with chicken bullion powder.	
B	**Savory Mushroom**: Double the amount of onion and sauté the onion with 8-16 ounces of fresh, sliced mushrooms. Delete the broccoli. Replace mushroom seasoning with 2 tsp thyme or Herbs de Provence.	

PROTEIN MEAT	**Balsamic Glazed Chicken** **Serves 3-4**	**Main**
INGREDIENTS		**SUBSTITUTE**
1-1½ lb	Boneless chicken breast	
1 Tbsp	Extra Virgin Olive Oil	Any olive or cooking oil
1 tsp	Minced garlic	½ tsp garlic powder
1 tsp	Salt (optional)	
2 tsp	Herbs de Provence	Oregano or any mix of oregano, basil, rosemary and thyme
¼ C	Balsamic vinegar	¼ C vinegar + 2 tsp any sugar or honey
4 oz	Goat cheese, crumbled	
STEPS		
1	Slice chicken breast into pieces ¼ - ½ inches thick.	
2	Toss sliced chicken with oil, garlic, herbs, and salt (if using).	
3	Sauté chicken over medium high heat until nicely browned and nearly cooked through.	
4	Reduce heat to medium low and add balsamic vinegar. Cook for a few minutes, turning chicken to coat. Vinegar should thicken and become syrupy.	
5	Serve chicken drizzled with the balsamic reduction from pan and top with crumbled goat cheese.	

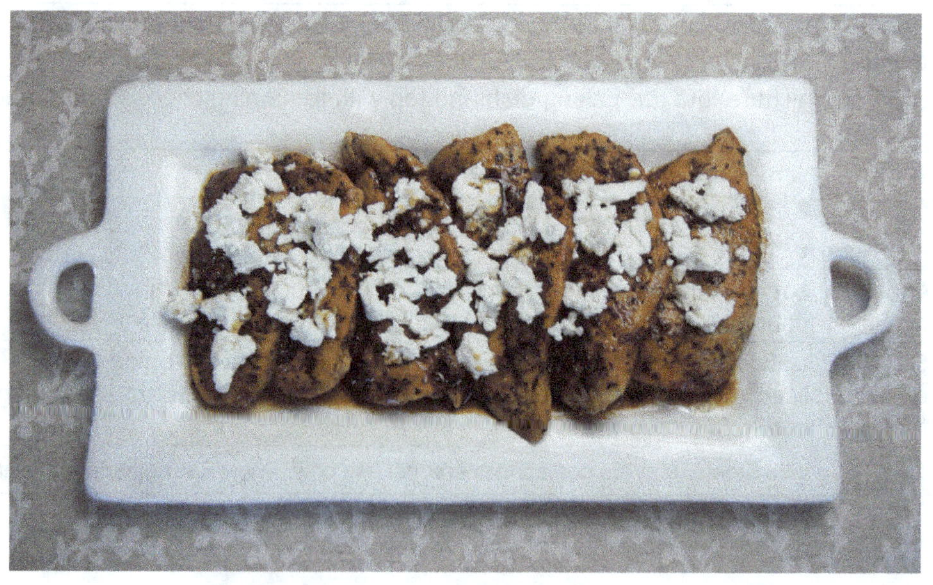

PROTEIN MEAT	**Beef Stroganoff** **Serves 4-6**	**Main**
INGREDIENTS		**SUBSTITUTE**
1-1½ lb	Beef steak, finely sliced	Lean ground beef
1	Onion, medium, finely sliced	
1 lb	Mushrooms, sliced (white or cremini)	
2 Tbsp	Extra Virgin Olive Oil	Any olive or light cooking oil
1 C	Sour cream	
1 tsp	Thyme	
1 tsp	Salt	
STEPS		
1	Sauté the onion and mushrooms in the olive oil over medium-high heat until the liquid has nearly completely evaporated.	
2	Stir in the sliced meat and continue to cook until the meat is just cooked through. Stir often so all sides of the meat are cooked. This should go quickly – maybe 2-3 minutes	
3	Remove from the heat and stir in the sour cream, thyme and salt.	
4	Serve with noodles, rice or potatoes.	

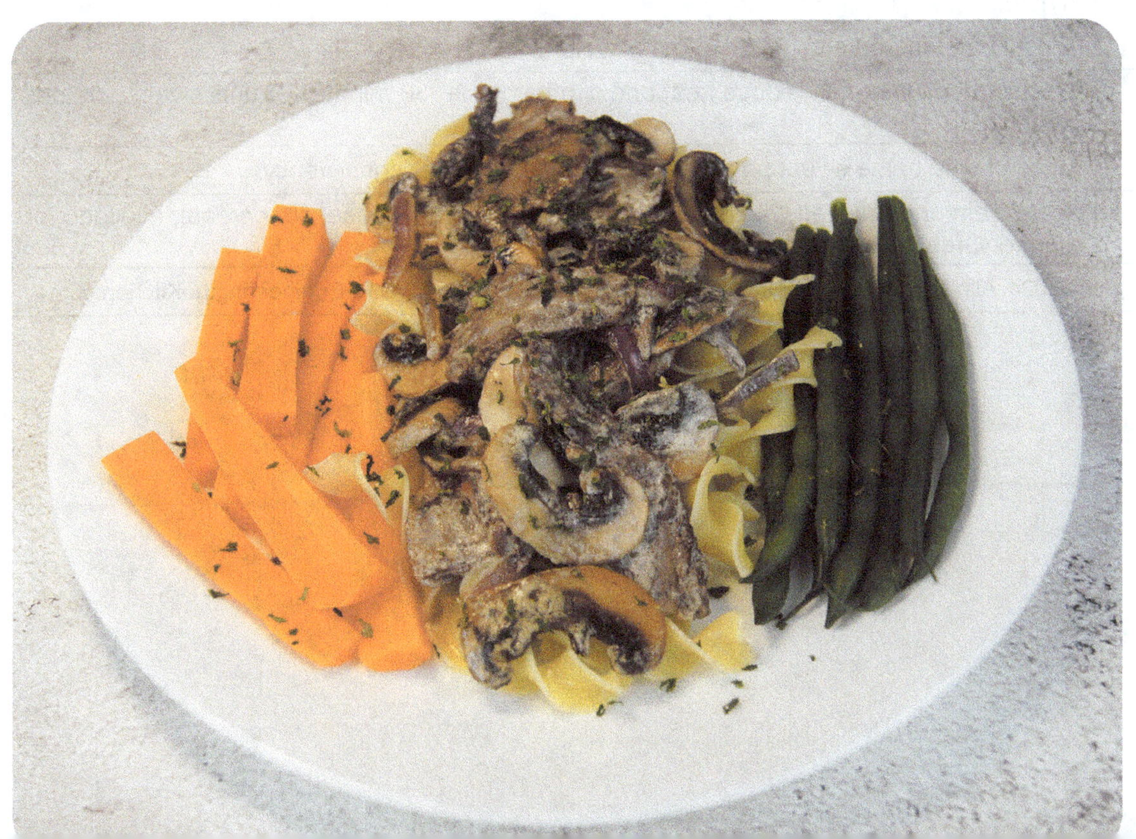

PROTEIN OTHER	Black Bean & Sweet Potato Chili[V] Serves 6	Main
INGREDIENTS		**SUBSTITUTE**
2 Tbsp	Extra Virgin Olive Oil	Any olive, coconut or other light cooking oil
1	Onion	
4	Cloves garlic	2 tsp minced jarred garlic
1½ Tbsp	Chili powder	
1 Tbsp	Cumin	
½ tsp	Paprika	
½ tsp	Oregano	
1	28 oz can diced tomatoes	Fire roasted or with green chilies
2	15 oz cans of black beans, drained	
1 lb	Sweet potatoes, diced (3-4 small)	Butternut squash
2 Tbsp	Lime juice	Lemon or orange juice
2 C	Vegetable or chicken stock	Water
STEPS		
1	In a large stock pot, sauté onion in the oil until soft. Add the garlic and cook for another 2 minutes.	
2	Add all other ingredients, stirring to mix well.	
3	Bring to a boil and then reduce heat and simmer for 20-30 minutes or until sweet potatoes are tender.	
4	Smash some of the sweet potatoes if you prefer a thicker consistency.	
5	Serve plain or garnished with diced red or green onions, cheese, sour cream, avocado, or cilantro. Great with steamed corn tortillas or corn bread.	

PROTEIN MEAT	Chicken Curry[V] Serves 3-5	Main
INGREDIENTS		**SUBSTITUTE**
2 Tbsp	Extra Virgin Olive Oil	Any olive oil, butter, Ghee or light oil
½	Onion, medium, diced	1½ Tbsp dehydrated onions
2	Garlic cloves, minced	1 tsp garlic powder or granules
2 -3 Tbsp	Curry paste	Any preferred curry spice paste
1-1½ lb	Chicken breast, cubed	Diced turkey, canned chicken
8 oz	Tomato sauce (1 can)	Diced tomatoes (blended, optional)
8 oz	Water	Broth or coconut milk
8 oz	Chopped spinach, frozen or fresh	Sweet potatoes (diced), peas or chickpeas
½ C	Cream	Yogurt or aerosol whipped cream

STEPS	
1	In a heavy bottomed sauce pan, sauté onion over medium heat until soft.
2	Add garlic and curry paste to pan and cook another two minutes.
3	Add tomato sauce and water to pan, stir and bring to a boil.
4	Reduce heat, add chicken and any desired veggies. Simmer for 15 minutes or until chicken is cooked and veggies are tender.
5	Remove from heat and stir in the cream.
6	Serve with rice, naan, paratha or cooked cauliflower.

OPTIONS	
A	**Vegetarian:** Replace chicken with two 15 oz cans of chickpeas (drained). Include one diced sweet potato and spinach if desired.
B	**Thickened:** For a thicker sauce, use a flour/butter paste. Mix 1 Tbsp each of flour & butter, then stir the paste ½ tsp at a time into the simmering sauce to reach desired consistency.

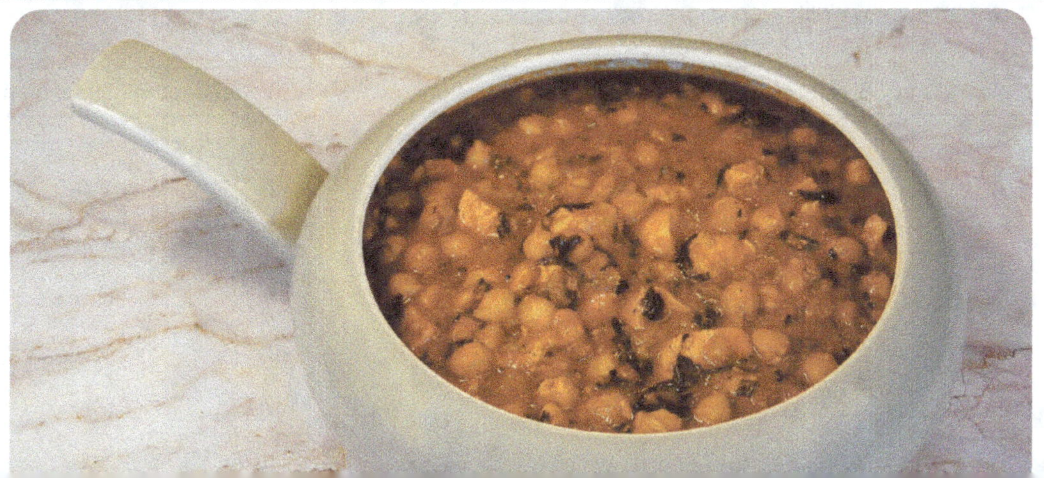

PROTEIN MEAT	**Chicken Divan** **Serves 2**	**Main**
INGREDIENTS		**SUBSTITUTE**
1 - 2	Cans chicken (6-12 oz total)	Any cooked and diced chicken or turkey
2 C	Chicken stock or broth	Bouillon cubes or stock paste + water
1 tsp	Dehydrated onions	2 Tbsp finely minced onions
⅓ C	Sherry	Any wine or 1 Tbsp of vinegar + 2 Tbsp water
2 Tbsp	Corn starch	
1 Tbsp	Mayonnaise	
1 Pkg	Broccoli spears, cooked and drained	Fresh or frozen
1 C	Shredded cheese (optional)	
½ C	Bread crumbs (optional)	Crushed crackers or unsweetened corn flakes
STEPS		
1	Warm chicken stock to almost boiling and add onions. Remove from heat.	
2	Stir corn starch into cold wine, mixing well.	
3	Stir wine and corn starch slurry into warm stock and return to heat. Warm over medium heat until thickened.	
4	Add chicken to thickened sauce and heat thoroughly over medium heat.	
5	Remove from heat and stir in mayonnaise.	
6	Can serve chicken and sauce over a bed of cooked broccoli.	
7	For a casserole, place brocolli and chicken in an oven proof casserole dish, top with cheese and/or bread crumbs. Bake for 10 minutes at 350°F for a crispy/melty top.	
OPTIONS		
A	**Nutritious Pantry Meal**: Serve alone for a quick and easy low-carb meal.	
B	**Extend the Meal**: Serve with rice, noodles, or grain to serve more people.	
C	**Complete Casserole**: Layer 2 C cooked rice or noodles wth brocolli and chicken mixture. Top with cheese and bread crumbs and bake for 20 minutes at 350°F.	

PROTEIN MEAT	**Chicken Mushroom Marsala** **Serves 3-6**	**Main**
INGREDIENTS		**SUBSTITUTE**
8-16 oz	Mushrooms, sliced	Frozen or canned mushrooms
1 tsp	Garlic, minced	½ tsp garlic granules
3 Tbsp	Olive oil	Any light oil
1-1½ lb	Chicken breast, sliced into thin cutlets	Veal or pork loin
½ C	Flour	
¾ C	Masala or Sherry (sweet wine)	Any red wine + 3 tsp sugar
½ Tbsp	Corn starch	
½ tsp	Salt and pepper, each	
STEPS		
1	Sauté mushrooms and garlic in 1 Tbsp of olive oil until mushrooms are cooked and most of the liquid is gone.	
2	Mix the corn starch into the cool wine then add to the mushroom pan. Stir over medium heat until the sauce thickens. Set aside and keep warm.	
3	Add salt and pepper to the flour in a shallow bowl.	
4	In a large skillet or sauté pan, heat the remaining 2 Tbsp of oil on medium heat until shimmering but not smoking.	
5	Dredge the chicken cutlets in the flour and place in the hot pan.	
6	Cook chicken until cooked through and lightly brown. Remove to platter.	
7	Serve chicken cutlets with mushroom and sweet wine sauce.	

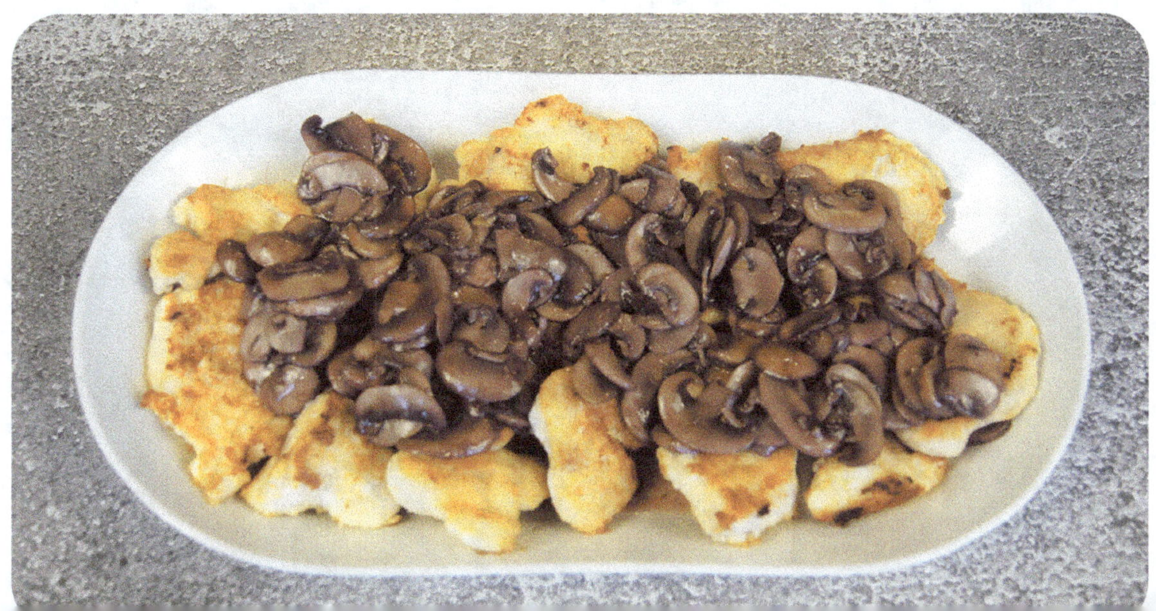

PROTEIN MEAT	**Chicken Paillard** **Serves 4-6**	**Main**
INGREDIENTS		**SUBSTITUTE**
1-1½ lbs	Boneless chicken breast	Chicken tenders or medallions
2 Tbsp	Extra Virgin Olive Oil	
1 tsp	Garlic, minced	Shallot or chives
2 Tbsp	Fresh thyme (2 tsp if dried)	Basil
2 Tbsp	Lemon juice (fresh is best) + lemon zest	White wine
¾ C	Chicken stock (used in optional sauce)	¾ C water + ¾ tsp bullion powder
	Salt and pepper to taste	

STEPS	
1	Slice each chicken breast into two or three cutlets, each ½ to ¾ inch thick.
2	Place cutlets one or two at a time, between sheets of plastic cling wrap. Use a meat mallet or rolling pin to pound the cutlets to half thickness.
3	Put pounded cutlets in a shallow dish and add the oil, lemon juice, and spices. Turn to coat and allow to rest for 15 minutes up to over night.
4	Reserve the residual marinade if you are making the optional sauce.
5	In a large sauté pan or skillet, pan fry the cutlets until golden on both sides. Use two pans or work in shifts so that the cutlets are not crowded in the pan.
6	Chicken cutlets may be served without optional sauce, for example on a green salad.
7	**Optional Sauce**: Add any remaining marinade and the chicken stock to the pan. Deglaze the pan over medium heat, stirring to fully incorporate. Cook a few minutes to allow sauce to thicken slightly. Drizzle over cutlets and serve.

PROTEIN MEAT	**Chicken Paprika** **Serves 2-4**	**Main**
INGREDIENTS		**SUBSTITUTE**
1½ -2 lb	Boneless chicken, thighs or breast	Bone-in chicken
1	Onion, large, diced	
1 Tbsp	Paprika	
1 tsp	Garlic, minced	½ tsp garlic powder or granules
8 oz	Tomato sauce	Diced tomatoes, canned or fresh
½ C	Sour cream	Yogurt
1 Tbsp	Flour	
	More paprika, salt and pepper to taste	

STEPS	
1	In a larger, heavy bottomed pot, sauté the onions with a little oil until soft. Add the garlic and paprika then cook an additional 2-3 minutes.
2	Add the chicken, tomato sauce and water to the pot.
3	Reduce heat, cover and simmer for at least 30 minutes. Chicken should be tender and cooked through.
4	Stir the flour into the sour cream, mixing well. Add this to the warm sauce and stir continuosly over low heat while the sauce thickens.
5	Serve with noodles, rice, potatoes or bread.

OPTIONS	
A	**Bone-in**: If you use pieces with skin and bones, then allow the chicken to simmer for 45 minutes to ensure it is thoroughly cooked.

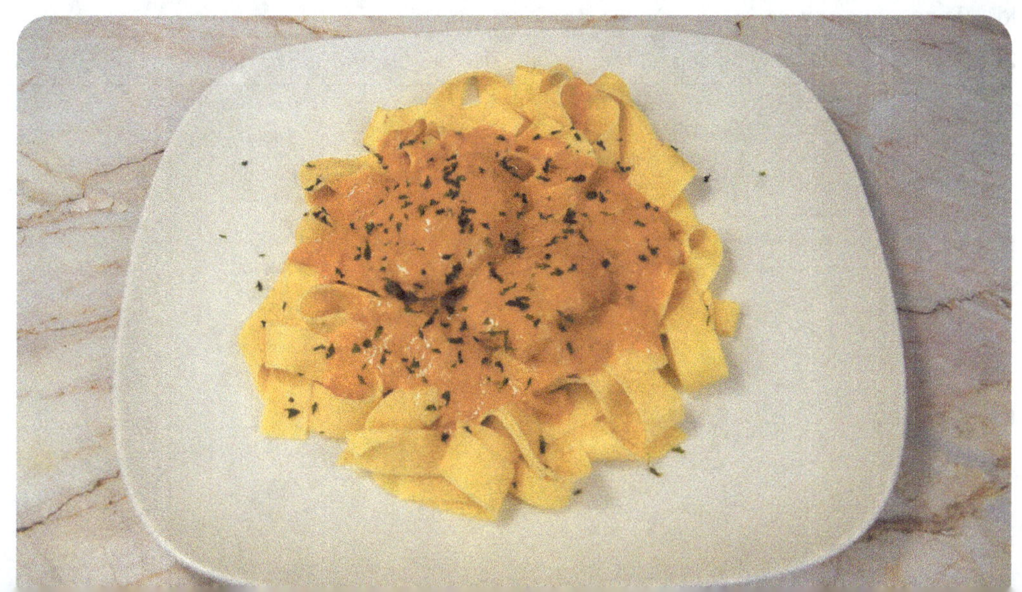

PROTEIN MEAT	Chicken Salad Serves 4	Main
INGREDIENTS		**SUBSTITUTE**
1 lb	Chicken breast, poached (see Poached Chicken recipe on page 114), diced	Any cooked chicken, cut up or shredded
¾ C	Mayonnaise	
¼ C	Sour cream	Yogurt
2	Green onions, finely sliced	2 Tbsp onion, finely minced
1-2	Celery stalks, finely diced	
1 tsp	Dijon mustard	
2 Tbsp	Fresh dill or tarragon	2 tsp dried dill or tarragon
2 Tbsp	Fresh parsley	2 tsp dried parsley
½ C	Seedless grapes, halved (optional)	Diced apples or dried cherries
¼ C	Slivered almonds (optional)	Chopped walnuts
STEPS		
1	In a large bowl, mix the mayonnaise, sour cream and Dijon mustard together.	
2	Add all remaining ingredients and stir to mix.	
3	Serve on bread, crackers or on a bed of greens.	
OPTIONS		
A	**Classic:** Recipe above.	
B	**Napa:** Include grapes and slivered almonds.	
C	**Cherry Chicken:** Include dried cherries and chopped walnuts.	
D	**Waldorf Chicken** Include grapes, apples and walnuts. Increase mayonnaise by ¼ C and add 1 Tbsp of honey.	

PROTEIN MEAT	**Chili Express** **Makes ~ 5 cups**	**Main**
INGREDIENTS		**SUBSTITUTE**
1 Tbsp	Extra Virgin Olive Oil	Any olive or light oil
1	Onion, medium, diced	3 Tbsp dry onion or 1 Tbsp onion powder
2	Cloves garlic, minced	1 tsp garlic powder or granules
1 lb	Ground turkey	Ground chicken or beef
1	Can (14.5 oz) cannellini beans, drained	Any canned beans
1	Can (14.5 oz) diced tomatoes (with chilis, optional)	Any canned tomatoes or sauce
1½ C	Chicken broth	1½ C water + 1/2 tsp bouillon or 1½ C water
2 Tbsp	Chili powder	
1 Tbsp	Cumin	
STEPS		
1	In a large heavy bottomed stock pot, sauté onion in oil until soft. Add garlic & cook for 1 min.	
2	Add turkey, chili powder and cumin. Cook over medium high heat, stirring to crumble turkey, until meat is cooked.	
3	Add tomatoes, beans and broth. For a less chunky result, the tomatoes may be blended first.	
4	Bring to a boil then reduce heat and simmer for at least 20 minutes.	
5	Serve alone or with with diced green onion, warm tortillas, corn bread, sour cream or melted cheese. Freezes well.	

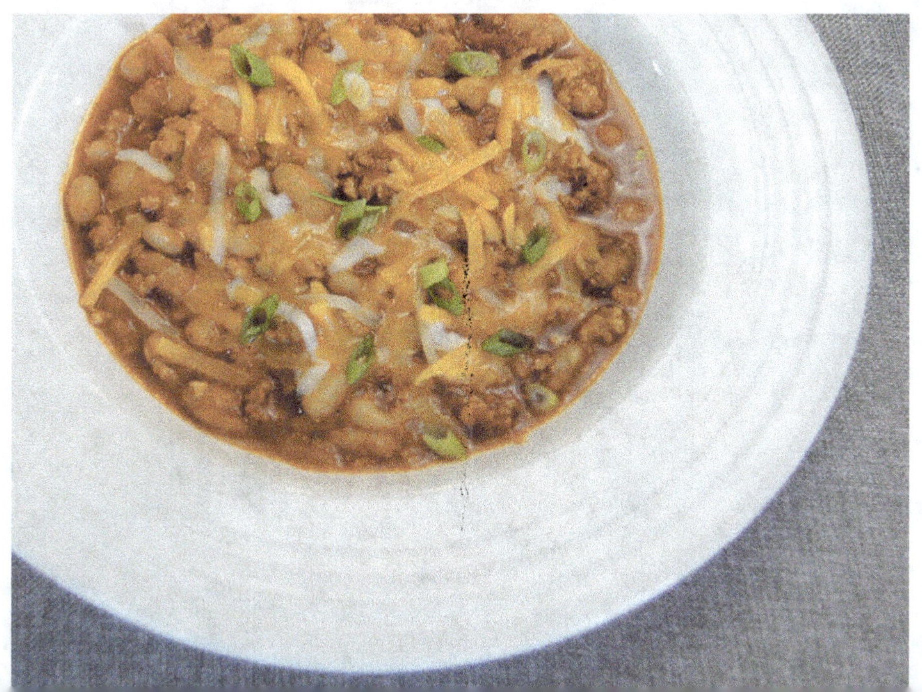

PROTEIN MEAT	**Citrus Grilled Shrimp** **Serves 2 - 4**	**Main**
INGREDIENTS		**SUBSTITUTE**
1 lb	Large shrimp or prawns	
1 tsp	Garlic powder	
1 tsp	Onion powder	
1 Tbsp	Chili powder	
1 Tbsp	Canola oil	Coconut oil or sesame oil
2 Tbsp	Orange juice concentrate	Orange juice
2 Tbsp	Grand Marnier	Any orange liquor or brandy
STEPS		
1	Rinse and devein shrimp. Remove tails if desired. Pat dry with a paper towel.	
2	Arrange shrimp in one layer on a plate. Apply half of the dry spices to one side, then flip and apply the rest to the other side.	
3	Heat oil in a large sauté pan – should be large enough that shrimp will fit in one layer.	
4	Over medium high heat, add the shrimp and cook for two minutes on one side. Flip and cook other side until shrimp is cooked: i.e. pink and not grey.	
5	Add orange juice and liquor to the pan, turning shrimp to coat and thicken sauce.	
6	Serve shrimp with rice, asian noodles, quinoa, or over salad greens.	

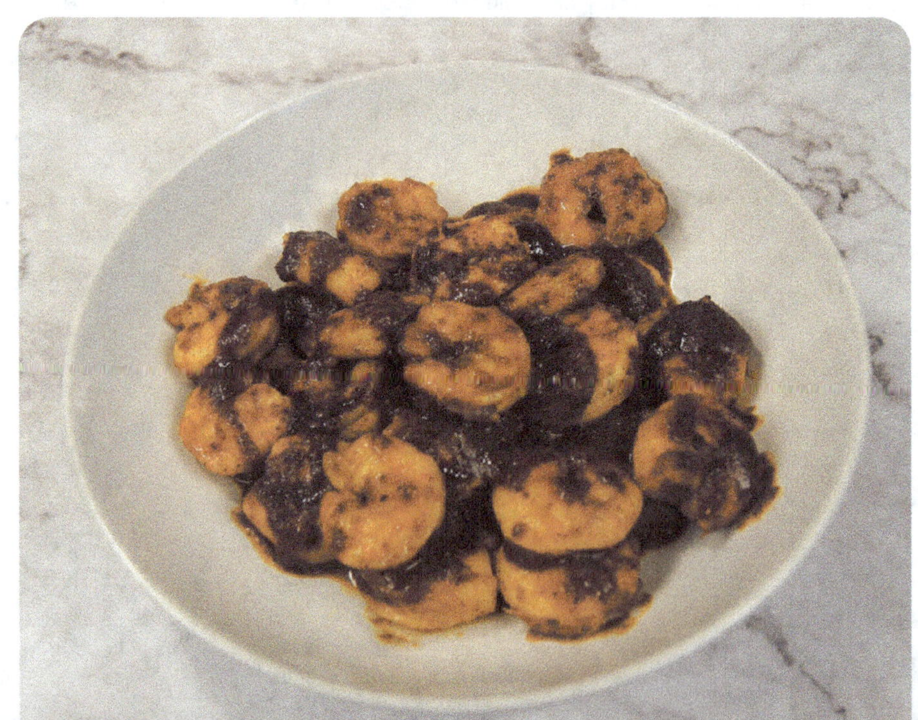

PROTEIN MEAT	**Crab Cakes** **Serves 4**	**Main**
INGREDIENTS		**SUBSTITUTE**
18 oz	Lump crab, canned and well drained	Fresh lump crab
1	Egg, large or larger	
3 Tbsp	Mayonnaise	Light mayonnaise
½ Tbsp	Dijon mustard	
1 tsp	Worcestershire	
1½ tsp	Old Bay seasoning	
1½ tsp	Lemon juice	
¾ C	Bread crumbs	Cracker crumbs
3 Tbsp	Melted butter (optional)	
STEPS		
1	Preheat oven to 400°F. Line a baking sheet with parchment paper.	
2	In a medium bowl, mix all ingredients except crab, crumbs and butter.	
3	Gently fold crab and crumbs into the egg-mayo mixture. Thoroughly distribute but avoid breaking up the lumps of crab.	
4	Chill the mixture for 30 minutes or more. This will make the mixture easier to form cakes.	
5	Form the crab mixture into 6 mounded cakes and place on the baking sheet. You can form the cakes by hand or by using a 1½ inch scoop. Each cake will be about ⅓ - ½ Cup.	
6	If desired, brush the crab cakes with melted butter for a crispier result.	
7	Bake for 15 minutes. Serve with slices of lemon or remoulade sauce.	
8	For an appetizer, make 18-24 mini crab cakes and bake for approximately 10 minutes.	

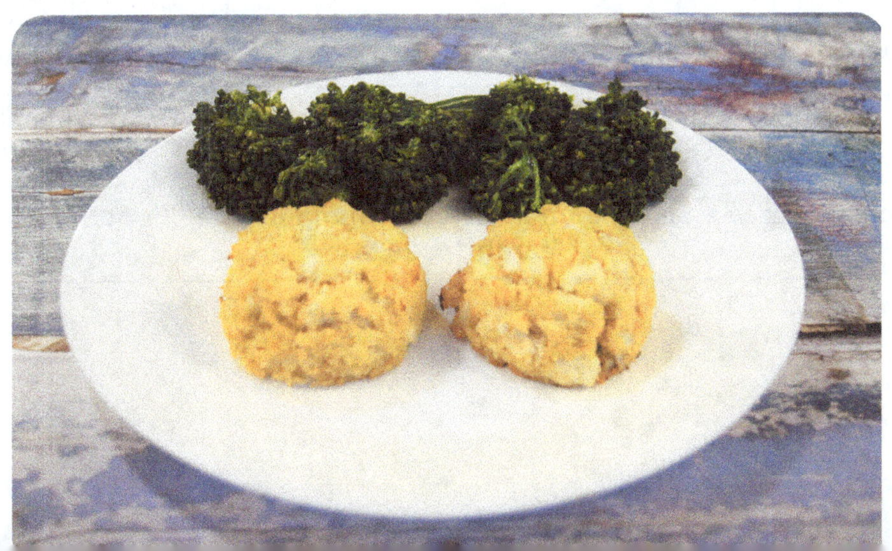

Safe Minimum Internal Temperature Chart for Cooking

Food	Type	Internal Temperature
Beef & Red Meats	Steaks, roasts, chops	145°F (63°C)
	Ground meat & sausage	160°F (71°C)
Poultry	Whole bird, breasts, legs, thighs, wings, ground, and sausage.	165°F (74°C)
Eggs	Raw eggs	Cook until yolk & white are firm
	Egg dishes (such as frittata or quiche)	160°F (71°C)
Ham	Raw ham	145°F (63°C) Rest time: 3 minutes
	Pre-cooked ham (reheat)	165°F (74°C)
Leftovers	Any type	165°F (74°C)
Pork	Steak, roasts, chops	145°F (63°C) Rest time: 3 minutes
	Ground meat & sausage	160°F (71°C)
Seafood	Fish such as salmon, tuna, cod, snapper, and sole	145°F (63°C) or cook until flesh is no longer translucent and separates easily with a fork
	Shrimp, lobster, crab, and scallops	Cook until flesh is pearly or white, and opaque
Source: Cook to a Safe Minimum Internal Temperature | FoodSafety.gov March 14, 2024		

PROTEIN MEAT	**Enchilada Surprise**[V] **Serves 4-6**	**Main**
INGREDIENTS		**SUBSTITUTE**
1	Medium onion, diced	
16	Corn tortillas	
16 oz	Grated cheese, Mexican blend	Co-Jack or mild cheddar or Queso Blanco
1	Can enchilada sauce (19 oz)	2-2½ C homemade Enchilada Sauce (see recipe on page 146)
½ -1 lb	Chicken, ground or diced	Beef, pork or turkey; precooked is OK.
1-2	15 oz cans black beans, drained	Other whole beans or refried beans
1	15 oz can corn, drained	½ bag of frozen corn, cooked and drained
1-2	Sweet potato, cooked and either mashed or diced	Canned sweet potato
STEPS		
1	Preheat oven to 350°F.	
2	If using uncooked meat, sauté onion and meat until meat is cooked through. For precooked meat, just add onion to the meat; it is fine to leave the diced onion uncooked.	
3	In a 9" x 9" pan (or 2½ quart casserole dish) just cover the bottom with sauce: about ⅓ cup. Place four tortillas on top of the sauce, spread out to cover the bottom.	
4	Spread one third of the meat, beans, corn and sweet potatoes over the tortillas, one-quarter of the cheese and then drizzle with one-third cup of sauce.	
5	Make the second layer with 4 tortillas then repeat step 4. Repeat to make the third layer.	
6	Use last four tortillas for the top layer, then cover with remaining sauce and then cheese.	
7	Bake for 30-45 minutes, until hot and bubbly. Serve with sour cream, green onion, avocado or salsa as desired.	
OPTIONS		
A	**Vegetarian**: Omit the meat and use black beans, corn and sweet potato for a delicious combination.	
B	**Tex-Mex**: Omit the sweet potatoes then use ground beef, corn, and red kidney beans or refried beans for a classic flavor.	
C	**Leftover Meat**: Use any precooked, diced meat including roast beef, chicken, pork or turkey.	
D	**Double Up**: Make a double recipe in a 9" x 13" pan.	

Photo on page 111

PROTEIN MEAT	**Fajitas** **Serves 4-6**	**Main**
INGREDIENTS		**SUBSTITUTE**
1½ - 2 lb	Steak - flank, skirt or other	Chicken breast, sliced horizontally, shrimp
¾ C	Fajita Marinade (recipe on page 119)	
2 Tbsp	Canola oil	
1	Onion, large, cut into slices	
2-3	Bell peppers, sliced (red, yellow and green)	
12	Tortillas, corn or flour	Naan, pita bread
STEPS		
1	Place the meat in a Ziploc bag or covered bowl with the Fajita Marinade and refrigerate for 2-24 hours. For shrimp, marinate for two hours.	
2	Ideally, grill the meat over a medium high fire to get nice caramelization on the outside. Steak takes about five minutes per side for medium rare. Chicken will take longer, shrimp less.	
3	Alternatively, use a large heavy skillet to cook the meat. Heat 1 Tbsp of the oil to shimmering and add the meat in one layer. Cook to desired doneness.	
4	Remove meat from the heat and allow to rest while cooking the vegetables.	
5	Add 1 Tbsp of oil to the heavy skillet, then cook the onions and peppers quickly over a medium high heat.	
6	Slice the meat into strips and serve with the vegetables and tortillas. Grated cheese, sour cream, salsa and guacamole compliment nicely.	

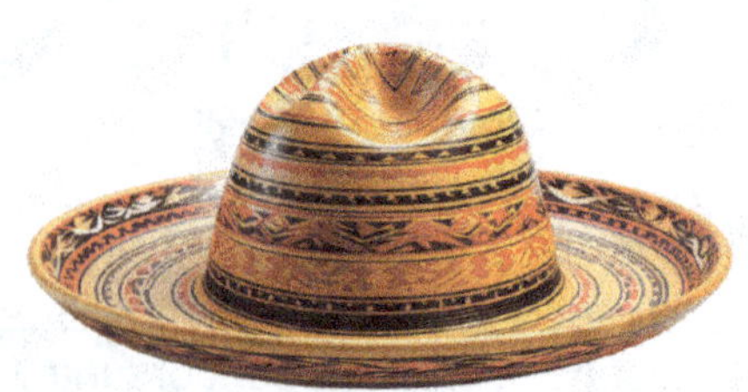

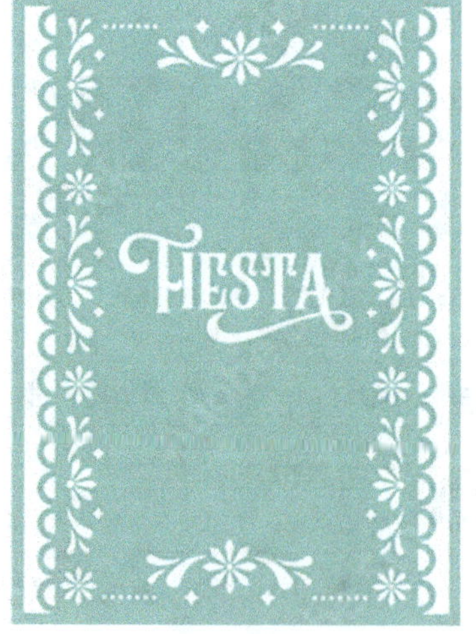

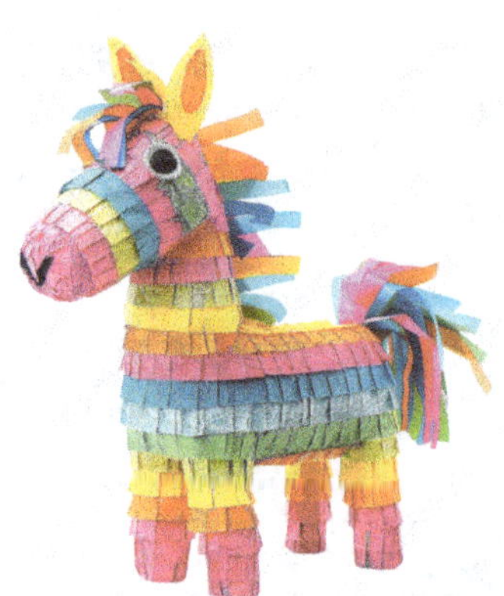

GRAIN	Fried Rice[V] Serves 2	Main
INGREDIENTS		**SUBSTITUTE**
2 C	Cooked rice, refrigerated day old preferred	
2 Tbsp	Canola oil	
3	Eggs, large or XL, beaten	
3	Green onions, sliced	
2	Carrots, diced, cooked	
1 Tbsp	Soy sauce	
1 tsp	Sesame oil	
1½ C	Peas, cooked	
4 oz	Cooked chicken or pork, diced (optional)	Firm tofu, diced, for vegetarian dish
STEPS		
1	Heat 1 Tbsp oil in a large skillet or wok. Pour in the eggs and stir to scramble.	
2	Once the eggs are set, add the rice and continue to cook over medium high heat, stirring to break up the rice and thoroughly mix.	
3	Push the eggs and rice to the side, add the remaining 1 Tbsp of oil and green onions to the middle. Cook for a minute then stir into the rice mixture.	
4	Add the cooked peas and meat (if using), along with the soy sauce and sesame oil to the pan. Continue to cook long enough to heat and mix.	

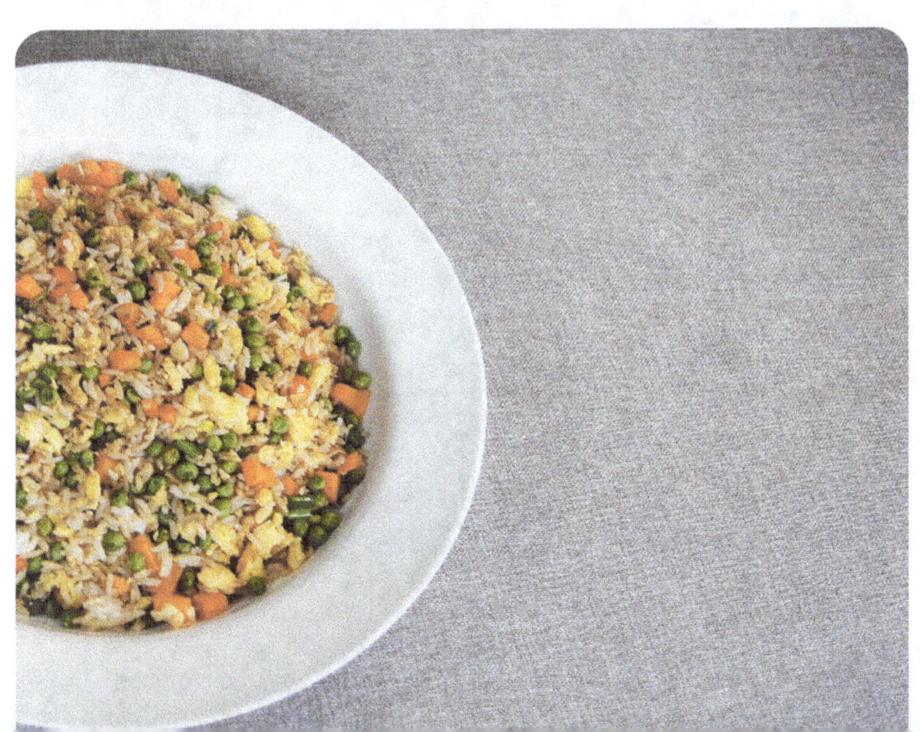

PROTEIN MEAT	**Hammered Chops** Serves 2-4	**Main**
INGREDIENTS		**SUBSTITUTE**
2 lbs	Pork chops, boneless	
½ C	Flour	
2 tsp	Garlic salt	Any savory spice blend
1 tsp	Black pepper	
¼ C	Oil – for pan frying	
STEPS		
1	Start with chops between ½ - ¾ inch thick. If your chops are thicker than this, slice them to get the right thickness.	
2	Place the chops one or two at a time between sheets of plastic wrap, on top of a cutting board.	
3	Using a meat mallet, pound the chops until they are about half the thickness.	
4	Mix the flour and spices in a shallow dish or container. Dredge each chop and set aside until ready to fry.	
5	In a large fry pan, heat the oil until shimmering but not smoking. Cook the chops in one layer until golden and cooked through, about 3 minutes per side.	
6	Cooked chops may be kept warm by placing them in one layer on a sheet pan in a 350°F oven until ready to serve.	

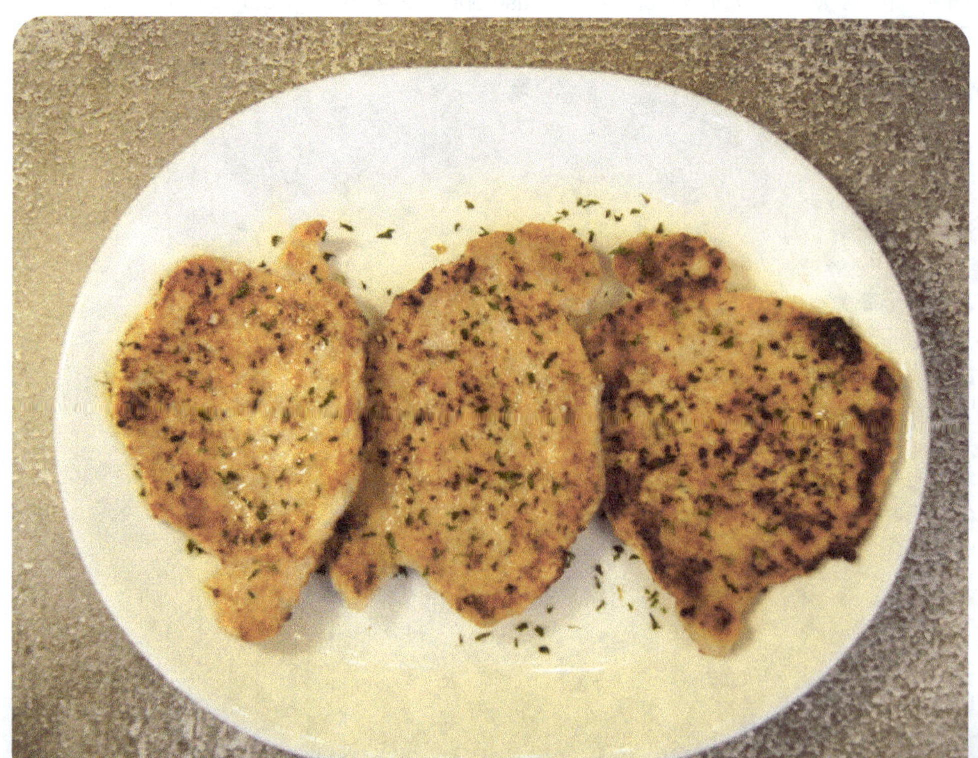

Dish in photo was made with 12 oz of pork, not the full recipe

PROTEIN MEAT	**Italian Sausage – Scratch** **Makes 1 lb**	**Main**
INGREDIENTS		**SUBSTITUTE**
1 lb	Ground pork	Ground turkey or chicken
1 Tbsp	Apple cider vinegar	Any vinegar or lemon juice
¾ tsp	Salt	
¾ tsp	Black pepper	
1½ tsp	Dried parsley	
2 tsp	Onion powder	
2 tsp	Garlic powder	
2 tsp	Oregano	
1 tsp	Paprika	
1 tsp	Fennel seeds, ground	
½ tsp	Thyme	
½ tsp	Basil	
½ tsp	Brown sugar	Any sugar or sweetener
¾ tsp	Red pepper flakes	For mild, use less or no red pepper flakes
STEPS		
1	In a bowl, mix ground meat with vinegar.	
2	Spread all dry spices over meat and mix until evenly distributed.	
3	For sausage logs, divide sausage into thirds and then form 1 inch diameter cylinders. Wrap cylinders in plastic wrap. (Skip this step if you want sausage crumbles.)	
4	Refrigerate 12-24 hours prior to cooking.	
5	Use as you would any uncooked italian sausage; e.g., spaghetti, lasagna, pizza.	

PROTEIN OTHER	**Lasagna Florentine**[V] **Makes two 9" x 13" pans**	**Main**
INGREDIENTS		**SUBSTITUTE**
6	Cloves garlic, minced	3 tsp jarred minced garlic
1 Tbsp	Extra Virgin Olive Oil	Butter
12 oz	Spinach, fresh, baby (8-16 oz)	Frozen spinach, thawed and drained
32 oz	Ricotta cheese	Cottage cheese, small curd
2	Eggs, large or XL	
48 oz	Marinara sauce	Store bought or use the Classic Marinara recipe on page 144
4 C	Mozzarella cheese, shredded (16 oz)	
2 ib	Lasagna noodles	Can use "oven ready" noodles
STEPS		
1	Sauté garlic in olive oil then add spinach and stir until just wilted.	
2	Mix ricotta cheese with eggs, then stir in spinach.	
3	Cook lasagna noodles until al dente, then drain and rinse. If using oven ready noodles, dip in sauce before putting them in the pan.	
4	In two 9"x13" greased pans, make four layers. The first three layers are sauce, noodles, ricotta, and mozzarella. The top layer is noodles, sauce and mozzarella.	
5	Cover pans tighly with greased foil. At this point, may be refrigerated for one day or frozen.	
6	Bake at 350°F covered for 45 minutes then for 15 minutes uncovered. (From frozen: 75 minutes covered then 10 minutes uncovered)	
7	Let stand for 10-15 minutes before slicing.	

PROTEIN MEAT	**Lemon Butter Baked Fish** **Serves 4**	**Main**
INGREDIENTS		**SUBSTITUTE**
4	Mild fish fillets, about 6 oz each, skinless	Cod, haddock, snapper, sole
6 Tbsp	Butter	
2 Tbsp	Lemon juice	
¾ C	Panko bread crumbs	Any bread crumbs, crushed crackers
1 Tbsp	Lemon pepper seasoning	
1 Tbsp	Dried parsley	
STEPS		
1	Preheat oven to 400°F.	
2	Melt 3 Tbsp of the butter in a shallow baking dish or pan, just big enough for your fillets. Add the lemon juice and stir.	
3	Melt the remaining 3 Tbsp of butter in a small bowl and mix in the seasoning, parsley and bread crumbs.	
4	Take each fillet and dip the top in the lemon butter then turn them over and place them in the pan.	
5	Top the fillets with the buttery crumb mixture.	
6	Cook for 20-25 minutes or until the fish has reached an internal temperature of 145°F.	

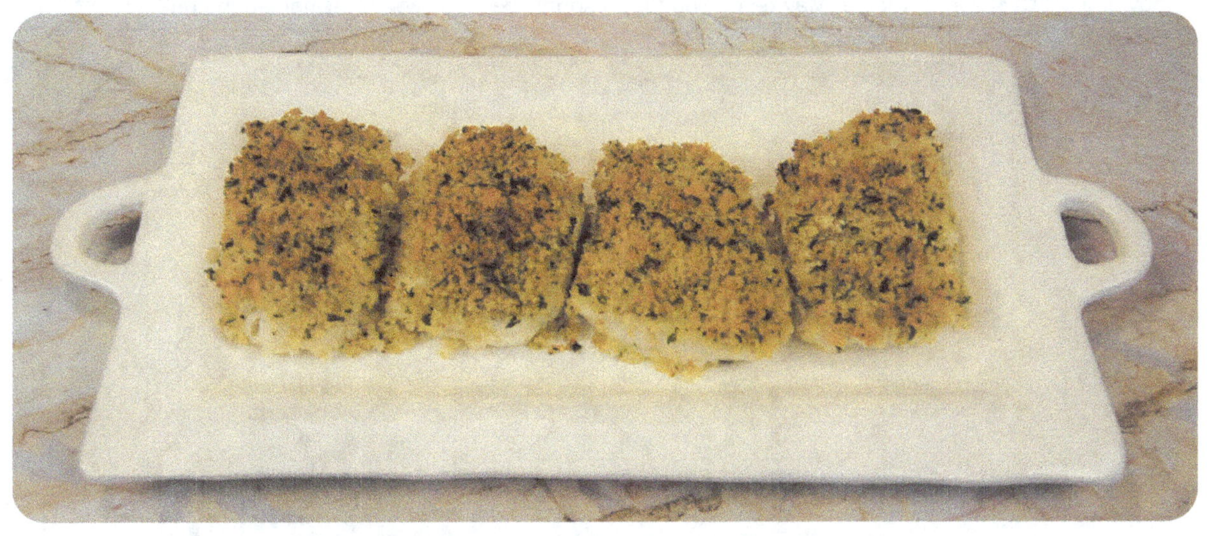

PROTEIN OTHER	**Lentils del Sol[V]** **Serves 2-4**	**Main**
INGREDIENTS		**SUBSTITUTE**
1½ C	Dry green lentils, rinsed	Any type of lentil
4 C	Chicken stock	Water
⅓ C	Sun dried tomatoes in oil, drained and diced	Dry sun dried tomatoes, soaked in hot water then finely sliced
⅓ C	Olive tepanade, prefer with Kalamata olives	⅓ C Kalamata olives + 2 cloves of garlic + 1 Tbsp olive oil, minced and combined
1-2 Tbsp	Extra Virgin Olive Oil	
2 tsp	Basil	Thyme or oregano
1 tsp	Salt	
1-2 Tbsp	Pine nuts (optional)	
STEPS		
1	In a large pot, bring lentils and stock to a boil. Reduce heat and simmer until lentils are tender but not mushy; 25-45 minutes depending on the type of lentil (refer to package).	
2	Drain any excess liquid from lentils. If you prefer your lentils less dry, leave about ½ C liquid in the pot.	
3	In a small bowl, mix the tomatoes, oil, tepanade, basil and salt together. Stir tomato and tepenade mixture into lentils.	
4	Cook over low heat for 5-10 minutes before serving as a main or side dish. Garnish with pine nuts if desired. Serve warm or cold. Makes about 4 cups.	

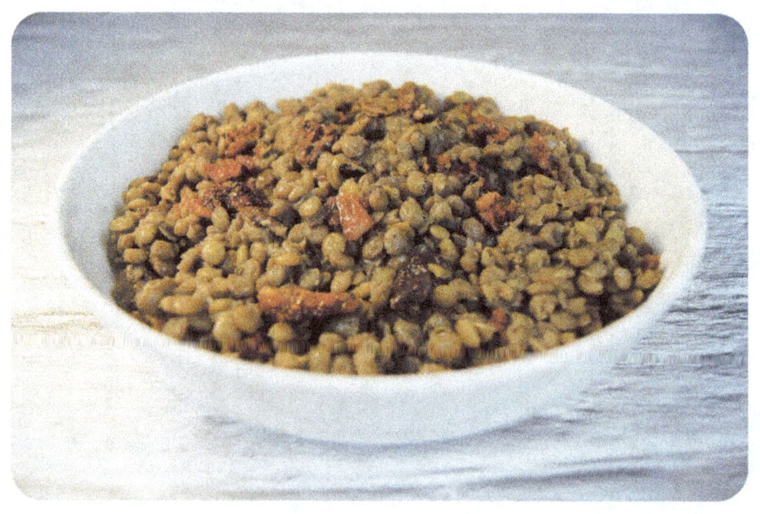

PROTEIN MEAT	**Marinated Flank Steak** **Serves ~ 6**	**Main**
INGREDIENTS		**SUBSTITUTE**
1	Flank steak (1½ - 2 ibs)	Skirt steak
½ C	Balsamic vinegar	Wine vinegar + 2 Tbsp sugar
2 Tbsp	Brown sugar	
2 tsp	Garlic, minced (fresh is best)	
2 tsp	Herbs de Provence	1 tsp Rosemary + 1 tsp Thyme
1 tsp	Salt	
½ tsp	Cracked black pepper	
STEPS		
1	Use a large fork to perforate steak on each side. This allow the marinade to penetrate the meat more effectively.	
2	Place meat in a gallon Ziploc bag (preferred) or a flat glass dish that may be covered.	
3	Mix marinade in a small bowl and then pour over the meat. Turn to ensure meat is covered.	
4	Allow to marinate over night, turning a few times to ensure even flavor.	
5	Take meat out of refrigerator an hour prior to cooking.	
6	GRILL METHOD: Preheat grill to Medium High. Grill steak on each side for 4-6 minutes. Internal temperature of 125 - 130°F will result in medium rare as temp will continue to rise.	
7	OVEN METHOD: Preheat oven to 425°F. Use a broiling pan and roast for 4-6 minutes per side. Internal temperature of 125-130°F will result in medium rare. Temp will continue to rise.	
8	Allow meat to rest for at least 5 minutes before carving.	
9	Cut meat into thin strips, slicing against the grain of the meat.	

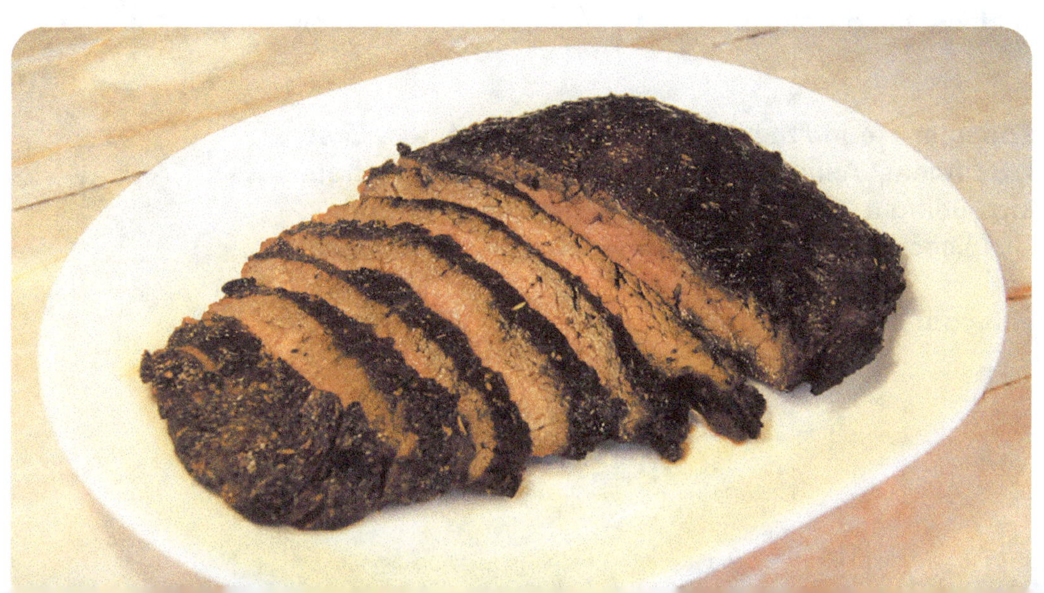

PROTEIN MEAT	**Meatballs – Italian** **Makes 8 - 12 meat balls**	**Main**
INGREDIENTS		**SUBSTITUTE**
1 lb	Ground beef	Ground pork, chicken, turkey, or lamb
2	Slices of bread, torn into pieces	½ C dried bread crumbs
3	Cloves garlic	1½ tsp minced jarred garlic
1	Egg, large or XL	
2 Tbsp	Milk	
¼ C	Grated Parmesan cheese	
2 tsp	Italian seasoning	Oregano or basil
STEPS		
1	Preheat oven to 400°F.	
2	Chop bread into crumbs using a blender or immersion blender. Add garlic cloves and blend until it is minced finely.	
3	In a bowl, mix all ingredients together until thoroughly incorporated. Can be done with hands, a large fork or a mixer.	
4	Form into uniform balls about 1½ inch diameter and place on baking sheet. An ice cream scoop works well to get a uniform shape and size.	
5	Bake for 15 minutes or until brown and cooked through (internal temperature of 160°F).	
6	Serve with you favorite sauce and pasta or to make meatball subs.	

Everyone, Almost Everywhere, Love Meatballs!

The first known reference to meatballs is in an ancient Roman collection of recipes, titled Apicius, which dates back to the 4th or 5th century CE.

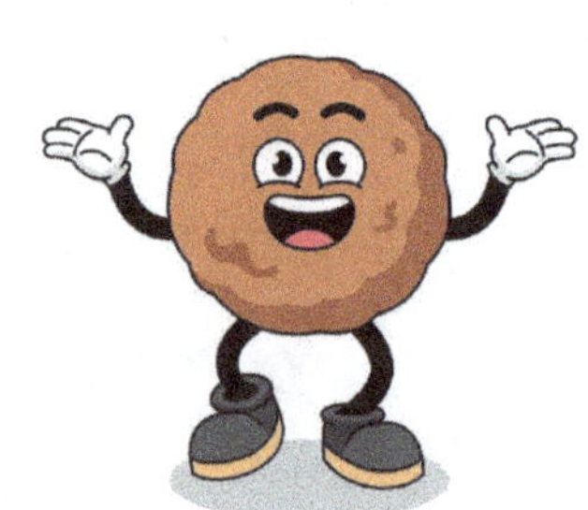

Meatballs are popular around the world - Europe, the Middle East, China, Japan, Southeast Asia, and the Americas. There are thousands of recipes using a large variety of meats, cheeses, grains, nuts, and local spices. Meatballs can be fried, baked, or steamed.

Experiment with your options and enjoy!

PROTEIN MEAT	**Meatloaf** **Serves ~ 8**	**Main**
INGREDIENTS		**SUBSTITUTE**
2 lb	Ground beef or beef-pork mixture	Any ground meat including chicken, turkey, pork, veal or lamb.
2	Medium onions, diced	⅓ C dried onions, soaked in 2 Tbsp hot water.
2	Eggs, large or XL	
2	Slices of bread, diced	½ C dry bread crumbs or rolled oats or crushed crackers or corn flakes
3 Tbsp	Worcestershire sauce	
2 Tbsp	Tomato paste	Ketchup
1 tsp	Salt and pepper, each	
1 tsp	Thyme or Herbs de Provence	Poutry seasoning may be used for ground chicken or turkey.
¼ C	Beef broth or bouillon	Use chicken broth for poultry.
½ C	Ketchup (can add some hot sauce if desired)	BBQ sauce or steak sauce
STEPS		
1	Preheat oven to 350°F.	
2	In a large mixing bowl, combine all ingredients except ketchup. Mix well but avoid compressing the mixture.	
3	Cover a sheet pan with foil or parchment paper for easier clean up (optional).	
4	Gently form the meat mixture into a rectangular loaf on the sheet pan. A 9 x 13 baking dish can be used but leave room around the loaf.	
5	Spread ketchup over the top of the loaf.	
6	Bake for 45-60 minutes, until the internal temperature reaches 165°F.	
OPTIONS		
A	**BBQ**: Substitute 1 tsp cumin and 1 tsp chili powder for thyme. Use BBQ sauce instead of ketchup on top. Add bacon crumbles if desired.	
B	**Italian**: Replace onions with 4-6 cloves of minced garlic and replace thyme with oregano. Spread marinara sauce on top instead of ketchup.	
C	**Mushroom**: Sauté 8-16 oz of sliced, fresh mushrooms then add to the meat mixture.	
D	**Cheeseburger**: Stir in 8 oz of diced or grated cheddar cheese. Use half steak sauce and half ketchup for the glaze.	

PROTEIN MEAT	**Oven-Fried Chicken** **Serves 4-6**	**Main**
INGREDIENTS		**SUBSTITUTE**
2 -3	Boneless chicken breast (1-1½ lb)	Chicken tenders or cutlets
¼ C	Mayonnaise	Any type, including reduced fat
½ tsp	Seasoning salt	
½ tsp	Black pepper	
1 tsp	Poultry seasoning	
½ tsp	Paprika	
1¼ C	Panko bread crumbs	Any dry bread crumbs, crushed corn flakes or crackers
STEPS		
1	Preheat oven to 400°F. Line sheet pan with parchment paper if desired.	
2	Slice chicken breasts into cutlets, medallions or strips which are ½ - ¾ inches thick.	
3	In a medium bowl, mix mayonnaise and spices. Add chicken pieces and turn to coat thoroughly.	
4	Put crumbs in a shallow bowl. Place one or two pieces of chicken at a time into the bread crumbs.	
5	Place breaded chicken pieces onto the sheet pan, leaving space between.	
6	For a crispier crust, lightly spray chicken with oil using an oil mister (optional).	
7	Bake for 20-25 minutes until chicken is cooked through (165°F in ternal temperature). Avoid overcooking as chicken will dry out.	
OPTIONS		
A	**Gluten Free**: Replace bread crumbs with almond meal or any unsweetened crispy crushed gluten free cereal made from corn, oats or rice.	
B	**Italian**: Use Italian seasoned bread crumbs and replace poultry seasoning with oregano or Italian seasoning.	
C	**Cajun Spicy**: Replace poultry seasoning and seasoning salt with a cajun spice blend. Add ¼ tsp red pepper flakes for extra heat.	
D	**Crispy Garnish**: Instead of discarding, stir remaining crumbs and mayo together then bake on the sheet pan along with the chicken. Use as a tasty crispy topping for a side dish.	

Photo on page 111

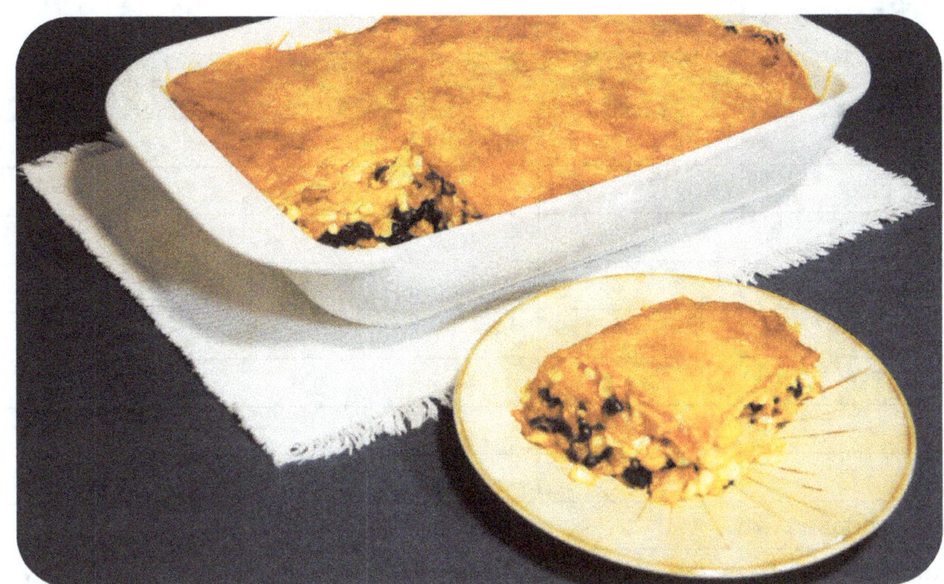

Enchilada Surprise

Recipe on page 99

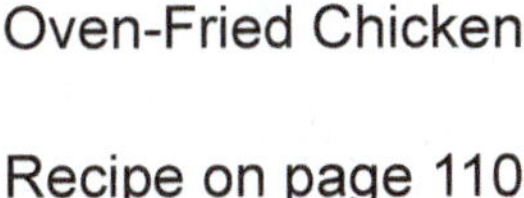

Oven-Fried Chicken

Recipe on page 110

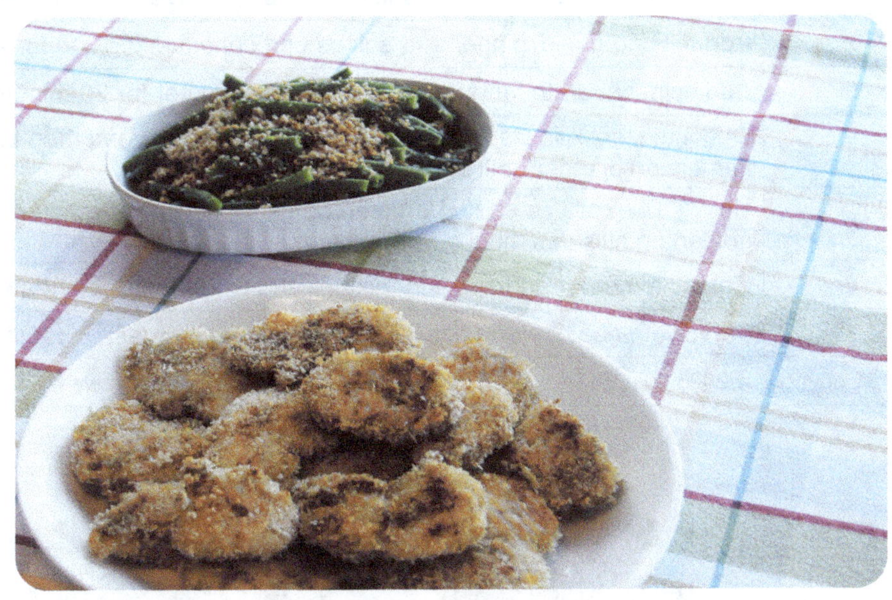

PROTEIN OTHER	**Palak Paneer** **Serves 4-6**	**Main**
INGREDIENTS		**SUBSTITUTE**
2 Tbsp	Extra Virgin Olive Oil	Any light cooking oil
1	Onion, medium, diced	
1 Tbsp	Garlic, minced	
2 Tbsp	Ginger root, grated	
1 Tbsp	Curry paste	Curry powder
2 tsp	Garam Masala	
2 tsp	Cumin	
2 tsp	Coriander	
16 oz	Spinach, frozen, chopped	
8 oz	Vegetable broth	Chicken broth or water
8 oz	Tomato sauce, canned	1 C diced fresh tomatoes
8-12 oz	Paneer, diced into small cubes	
STEPS		
1	In a heavy sauté pan, sauté onion in 1 Tbsp oil over medium heat until soft.	
2	Add minced garlic, ginger and spices and continue cooking for an additional three minutes.	
3	Add spinach, broth, and tomato sauce and simmer for 20 minutes.	
4	Optional step: Allow spinach mixture to cook slightly and then blend in a blender or with an immersion blender until smooth.	
5	Heat 1 Tbsp oil in a sauté pan (can be same pan) over medium heat and brown paneer until golden on all sides, about 5 - 7 minutes.	
6	Combine paneer and spinach mixture and warm until well heated.	
7	Serve with rice or warm naan (or paratha) or with roasted cauliflower or cauliflower rice.	

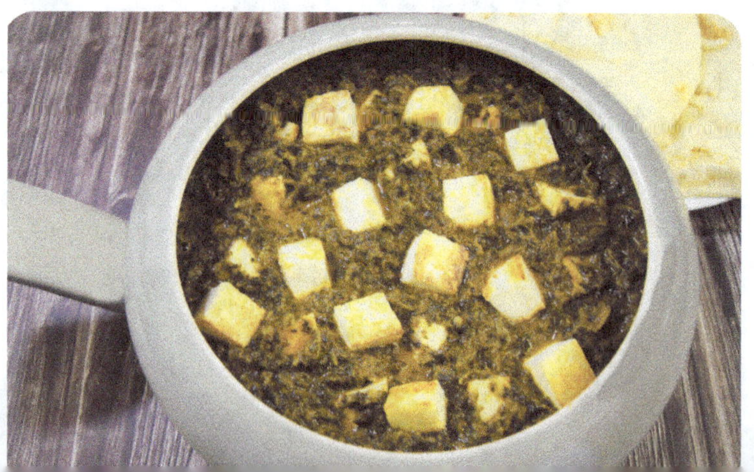

PROTEIN MEAT	**Picadillo** **Serves 4-6**	**Main**
INGREDIENTS		**SUBSTITUTE**
1 lb	Ground beef	Half ground pork + half ground beef
2	Onions, medium, chopped	
2	Cloves garlic, minced	
2 Tbsp	Extra Virgin Olive Oil	Any olive oil or light cooking oil
1	15 oz can of tomatoes, diced or crushed	
1 tsp	Oregano	
1 Tbsp	Vinegar	
½ C	Raisins, chopped	
1 Tbsp	Tomato paste	2 Tbsp ketchup (omit vinegar)
½ C	Green olives with pimento, sliced or whole	
STEPS		
1	In a large heavy bottomed pot, sauté onion in oil until soft then add the garlic and cook for an additional two minutes.	
2	Add ground beef and brown. Drain excess oil if necessary.	
3	Add remaining ingredients and bring to a boil.	
4	Reduce heat, cover and simmer for about an hour. Stir occasionally.	
5	Serve with white rice and black beans, or moro (recipe on page 298).	

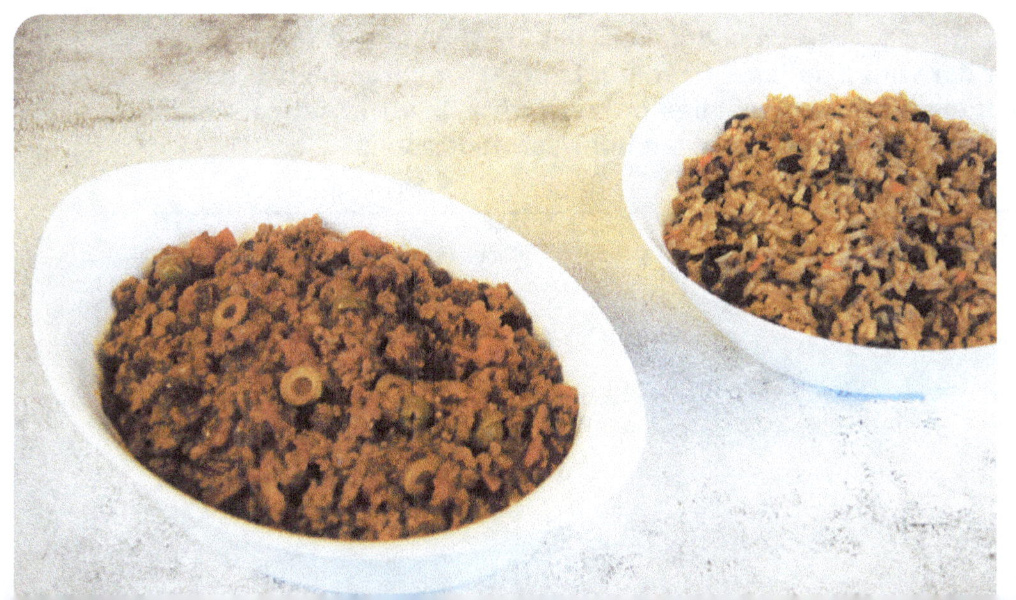

Shown with Cuban Moro Beans & Rice

Recipe on page 154

PROTEIN MEAT	Poached Chicken Serves ~ 2	Main
INGREDIENTS		**SUBSTITUTE**
2-4	Chicken breast, whole, boneless	Fish fillets, shellfish
	Water	Chicken broth
	Lemon (optional)	Garlic
	Herbs de Provence (optional)	Rosemary, Italian seasoning
STEPS		
1	Select a pot with a tight-fitting lid, large enough that the chicken breast fit snugly in a single layer.	
2	Place the chicken breasts in the pot and add any desired flavorings such as lemon, garlic or herbs.	
3	Cover chicken breast with enough water to cover the chicken breast plus two inches.	
4	Bring the liquid to a boil over medium high heat. Immediately turn the heat down to a simmer and cover the pot.	
5	Simmer for 10-15 minutes, until the internal temperature reaches 165°F. Start checking the temperature after about 10 minutes. For seafood, reduce time as needed.	
6	Remove chicken from the liquid and allow to stand for five minutes prior to slicing. If not using immediately, store chicken uncut to maintain moisture.	
7	Poached chicken is great in salads, casseroles, sliced for sandwiches or served sliced with a complimentary sauce.	

Why poach?

Poaching is a great way to cook chicken, fish or shellfish so that it stays moist and tender with a delicate flavor. It is ideal for serving chicken or seafood cold; in salads, sandwiches or just with a flavorful sauce. Poaching is also a great way to quickly cook an item before it spoils!

PROTEIN MEAT	**Roast Pork Tenderloin** **Serves 6-10**	**Main**
INGREDIENTS		**SUBSTITUTE**
2	Pork tenderloins, about 2½ lbs	
1 recipe	Apple Cider Vinegar Marinade (page 128)	Dry rub, BBQ sauce
STEPS		
1	Make the marinade in a gallon Ziploc bag and add the pork. Allow pork to marinate overnight in the refrigerator, turning occasionally.	
2	Preheat oven to 400°F.	
3	Place tenderloins on a broiling pan or roasting pan, preferably with grates or a rack.	
4	Roast for 30-40 minutes. Test for doneness with an instant read thermometer inserted in the thickest part of the meat. An internal temperature of at least 145°F is recommended.	
5	Allow the pork to rest for at least 5 minutes before slicing and serving.	
OPTIONS		
A	**Dry Rub**: Instead of marinating the pork, simply coat the exterior with your favorite spice blend or dry rub.	
B	**BBQ**: Instead of marinating the pork, brush the top with your favorite BBQ sauce once before putting it in the oven and again after 20 minutes.	

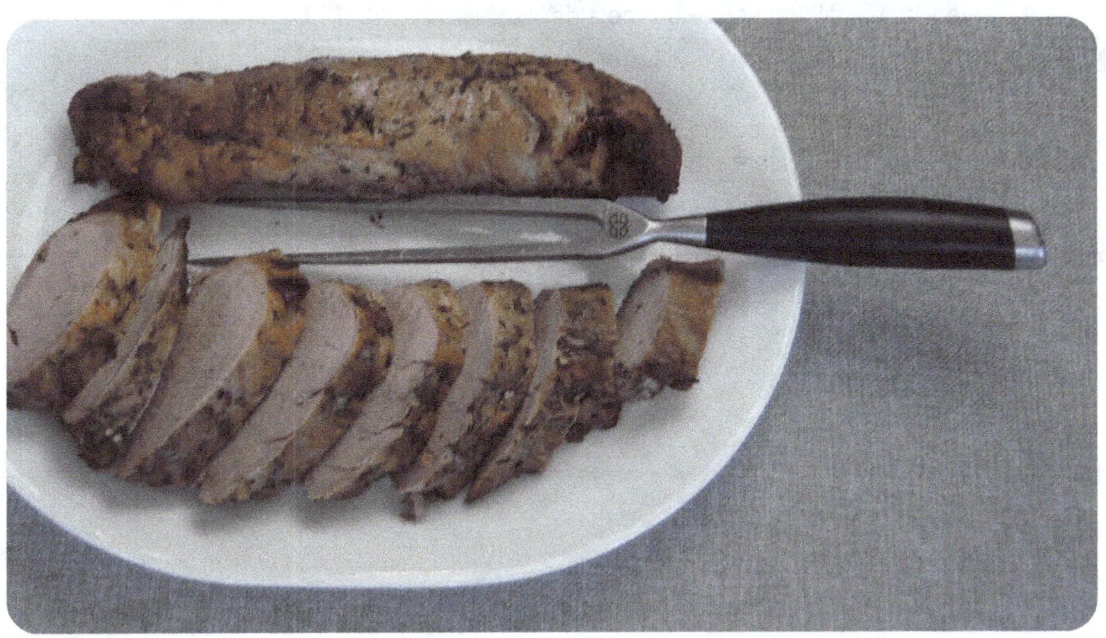

PROTEIN MEAT	**Salmon with Sweet Mustard Glaze** **Serves 4**	**Main**
INGREDIENTS		**SUBSTITUTE**
4	Salmon fillets, 6-8 oz each	Skin on or skinless, fresh or previously frozen
4 Tbsp	Brown sugar	
1 tsp	Ginger paste	1 tsp dried ginger
2 Tbsp	Dijon mustard	
2 Tbsp	Soy sauce	
STEPS		
1	Preheat oven to 400°F. Prepare baking pan or sheet pan by coating with oil.	
2	Prepare the salmon by removing any bones, rinsing and then patting dry.	
3	Mix the remaining ingredient together which will form both the glaze and a dipping sauce.	
4	Place the fillets in the pan and brush half of the mixture on top of the fillets.	
5	Bake for about 10-15 minutes until desired doneness. An internal temperature of 135°F for medium and 145°F for well done.	
6	If you would like a crispy upper crust, you can turn on the broiler for 3-5 minutes.	
7	Once cooked, the flesh may be easily separated from the skin by slipping a very thin metal spatula between them.	
8	Serve with remaining sauce on the side.	
OPTIONS		
A	**Citrus Glazed**: Replace the soy sauce, Dijon, and ginger with 2 Tbsp orange juice concentrate and ½ tsp each salt and paprika. Use all glaze.	
B	**Blackened**: Replace the soy sauce, ginger, Dijon, and brown sugar with 2 Tbsp Cajun seasoning mix. Use all to glaze. For a sweeter result, include 2 Tbsp of the brown sugar.	

Photo on page 127

PROTEIN MEAT	Shrimp & Cheesy Grits Serves 4	Main
INGREDIENTS		**SUBSTITUTE**
1 C	Old Fashioned Grits	Quick or instant grits work if necessary but are not prefered
6 oz	Sharp cheddar cheese, grated	
2 oz	Mild cheddar, colby or cojack cheese, grated	
1 lb	Shrimp, peeled and deveined	
2 Tbsp	Cajun spice blend	
1-2 Tbsp	Canola oil	Any light cooking oil
2 Tbsp	BBQ sauce	
2 Tbsp	Sliced green onions for garnish (optional)	Parsley
STEPS		
1	Prepare grits to package instructions.	
2	Stir in grated cheese and allow to melt. May be made ahead of time and reheated.	
3	Pat clean shrimp dry with a paper towel. Arrange in a flat layer on a plate.	
4	Sprinkle 1 Tbsp of the Cajun spice blend on the shrimp. Flip shrimp over and apply the rest of the spice blend to the other side.	
5	In a large fry pan, heat the oil over a medium high heat until it shimmers.	
6	Add the shrimp and cook on one side for 2 minutes. Flip the shrimp over and cook for an additional 2 minutes until just cooked through. Shrimp should be pink and form a "C" shape.	
7	Quickly add the BBQ sauce and shake the pan to coat the shrimp.	
8	Serve immediately over warm, cheesy grits and garnish with green onion if desired.	

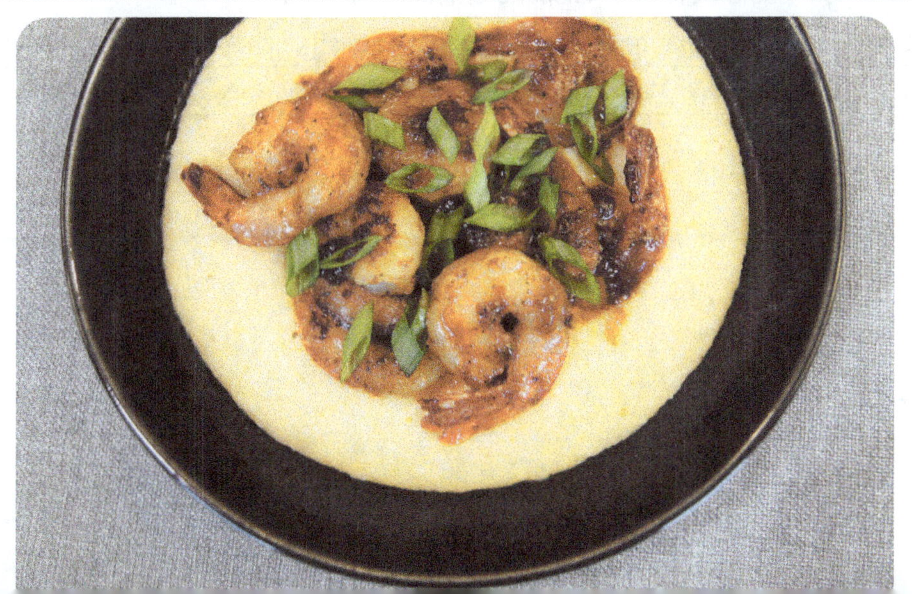

PROTEIN MEAT	**Shrimp Scampi** **Serves 4**	**Main**
INGREDIENTS		**SUBSTITUTE**
12 oz	Angel hair pasta	Linguini
1 lb	Shrimp, cleaned and deveined	
4	Cloves garlic, minced	2 tsp jarred minced garlic
2 Tbsp	Extra Virgin Olive Oil	
1 C	Dry white wine	
3 Tbsp	Lemon juice	
5 Tbsp	Butter	
1 tsp	Salt	
¼ tsp	Red pepper flakes (optional)	
½ C	Grated parmesan cheese	
2 Tbsp	Fresh parsley, garnish (optional)	
STEPS		
1	Cook the pasta to slightly less than al dente. It will cook more later. Reserve 1 C of the pasta water.	
2	In a large pan, heat the olive oil and add the garlic. Cook for about one minute.	
3	Cook the shrimp until it is just cooked through, about two minutes per side. Using a slotted spoon, remove the shrimp to a plate.	
4	Add the wine, lemon juice, salt, and red pepper flakes to the pan and cook for three minutes to allow sauce to thicken slightly.	
5	Add the shrimp back to the pan, along with the pasta, butter and ¼ C pasta water. Cook while turning in the pan to coat the pasta and melt the butter.	
6	Add more pasta water in 2 Tbsp increments if needed.	
7	Serve topped with parmesan cheese and a garnish of chopped fresh parsley.	

Photo on page 127

PROTEIN MEAT	**Sloppy Joes** Serves ~ 4	**Main**
INGREDIENTS		**SUBSTITUTE**
1-1¼ lb	Ground beef	Ground turkey or ground chicken
½	Onion, medium diced	1½ Tbsp dried onion or ½ Tbsp onion powder
1	Red bell pepper	Green or yellow pepper
1 tsp	Garlic, minced	½ tsp garlic powder or granules
¾ C	Ketchup	[1/2 C tomato paste + 1 tsp sugar + 1 Tbsp vinegar + ¼ C water] or [8 oz tomato sauce + 1 tsp sugar + 1 Tbsp vinegar]
2 Tbsp	Brown sugar	Any sweetener
1 tsp	Mustard, yellow or Dijon	1 tsp dry mustard powder
½ C	Water	
1 tsp	Corn starch	
½ tsp	Salt and pepper, each	
STEPS		
1	Brown meat, onion and garlic in large frying pan. Drain excess oil if necessary.	
2	Add ¼ C water, ketchup, sugar, and mustard to the pan then bring to a boil.	
3	Reduce heat and simmer for 5-10 minutes, stirring occasionally.	
4	Mix corn starch and ¼ C cool water together. Add to pan over low heat and stir until thickened. Salt and pepper to taste.	
5	Serve on hamburger buns, dinner rolls for sliders or over rice or cauliflower rice.	

PROTEIN MEAT	**Spaghetti Sauce** Serves 6-10	**Main**
INGREDIENTS		**SUBSTITUTE**
1 lb	Ground beef, lean	Ground turkey, chicken or pork
2 Tbsp	Extra Virgin Olive Oil	Any olive or light oil
1	Onion, diced	
2	Cloves garlic, minced	1 tsp minced jarred garlic
1 Tbsp	Flour	
1 C	Dry red wine	Any dry wine
28 oz	Can crushed tomatoes	Diced tomatoes or whole tomatoes cut up
6 oz	Tomato paste	
1 C	Beef broth	Water + bouillon powder
2 tsp	Oregano	Basil or Italian Seasoning
1 C	Mushrooms, fresh sliced (optional)	Canned mushrooms
STEPS		
1	In a stock pot, sauté onion in the oil until soft. Add the garlic and cook for an additional minute.	
2	Stir the flour into the ground beef and then add it to the pot and cook until crumbly.	
3	Add the wine and cook over medium high heat for two minutes.	
4	Add remaining ingredients and simmer over low heat, stirring occasionally. If you are in a rush, simmer for a half hour but simmering for 1½ hours will produce a better flavor.	
5	Serve with pasta or any dish calling for a tomato based Italian sauce. Freezes well.	

PROTEIN OTHER	**Stuffed Shells^{V}** **Serves 4-6**	**Main**
INGREDIENTS		**SUBSTITUTE**
16 oz	Ricotta cheese	
2	Eggs, large or XL	
3 Tbsp	Grated Parmesan cheese	Grated mozzarella, Romano, or Swiss cheese
1 box	Jumbo shells, uncooked	
6 C	Chicken broth or vegetable stock	6 C water + 6 tsp bullion powder
	Olive oil and grated cheese for serving	Alfredo sauce, marinara sauce, or sour cream
STEPS		
1	In a medium sized bowl, mix the ricotta cheese, eggs and grated Parmesan well.	
2	Fill uncooked shells with the ricotta mixture. Set the filled shells aside on plates or a cookie sheet. You will use about 24 shells.	
3	Place two large (10 inch diameter) skillets or stock pots with tight-fitting lids on the stove and put half of the broth in each one. Bring liquid to a boil.	
4	Turn off heat and carefully place half of the shells in each of the pots, open side facing up. A large spoon or tongs work well. Shells should be almost submerged.	
5	Turn heat back on to a gentle simmer and place the lids on the pots. Check that the liquid does not boil too vigorously as this will dislodge the cheese from the shells.	
6	Cook for 15-20 minutes, until shells are cooked to al dente.	
7	Remove cooked shells to a serving dish with a slotted spoon, gently draining any residual liquid.	
8	Serve plain or with your choice of topping such as butter or olive oil and grated cheese, sour cream, Alfredo sauce, or Marinara sauce.	

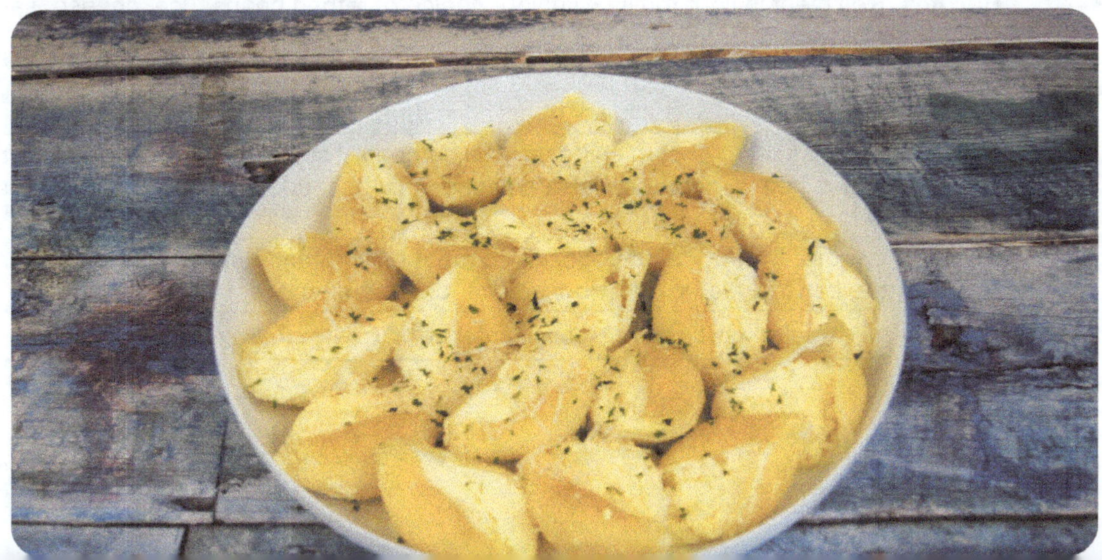

PROTEIN MEAT	Tacos Serves 3-4	Main
INGREDIENTS		**SUBSTITUTE**
1	Medium onion, diced	2 Tbsp dehydrated onion
1 lb	Ground beef	Any ground or diced meat: chicken or turkey
2	Cloves garlic, minced	1 tsp jarred garlic or ⅔ tsp garlic powder
1½ Tbsp	Chili powder	
1 Tbsp	Cumin	
½ tsp	Oregano	
½ tsp	Paprika	
1 tsp	Salt	
1 tsp	Sugar	
2 Tbsp	Tomato paste	Ketchup (eliminate sugar)
2 tsp	Corn starch	
½ C	Beef broth (cold)	Chicken broth or just water
STEPS		
1	Sauté onion in an oiled pan until soft. (If using dehydrated onion, just add it to meat.)	
2	Add garlic and ground meat to pan. Brown over medium heat.	
3	Skim off excess fat if necessary.	
4	Add all spices and tomato paste, then mix well. Allow to cook for about 5 minutes.	
5	Mix corn starch into broth until smooth. Add to meat & stir over medium heat until thickened.	
OPTIONS		
A	**Tacos:** Serve in corn or flour tortillas with cheese, lettuce, tomato, salsa, sour cream, etc.	
B	**Burritos**: Roll meat in flour tortilla with your choice of refried beans, rice, cheese, salsa, etc.	
C	**Taco Pie** - Mix meat with 1 bag of cooked frozen corn and place in the bottom of a baking dish. Top with 1 package of corn bread dough made to package instructions and then bake for 15-20 minutes at 350°F or until corn bread is done.	
D	**Nachos**: Spread a layer of corn chips on a baking pan. Top chips with meat mixture and choice of refried beans, peppers, salsa and cheese. Toast under broiler to melt cheese (or 400°F oven for 5 minutes).	
E	**Stuffed Peppers**: Fill any clean pepper with meat mixture and bake at 350°F for 45 minutes. Meat mixture can include up 50% cooked rice, drained beans, or corn.	

PROTEIN MEAT	Teriyaki for All Serves 4-6	Main
INGREDIENTS		**SUBSTITUTE**
2 lb	Chicken breast or thighs, boneless, skinless	Boneless steak or pork, or shrimp
1 C	Teriyaki Marinade (recipe on page 129)	
⅓ C	Water (cold)	
2 tsp	Corn starch	
1 Tbsp	Canola oil	
1 tsp	Sesame oil (optional)	
	Green onions and sesame seeds for serving	
STEPS		
1	Cut meat into one inch pieces and put into Ziploc bag or covered dish.	
2	Pour ⅔ C of the teriyaki marinade over the meat and refrigerate for two to six hours. Reserve the remaining ⅓ C marinade for later.	
3	After the meat has marinated, remove it from the marinade and discard the used liquid.	
4	In a large skillet, heat the canola oil to shimmering and add the meat. Cook the meat quickly over medium high heat.	
5	Mix the reserved marinade with the water, corn starch and sesame oil (if using), stirring to form a smooth slurry.	
6	When the meat is thoroughly cooked, add the marinade/cornstarch mixture and cook for 3-5 minutes while stirring. The sauce should thicken and coat the meat.	
7	Serve with rice and veggies, garnished with sliced green onions and sesame seeds as desired.	

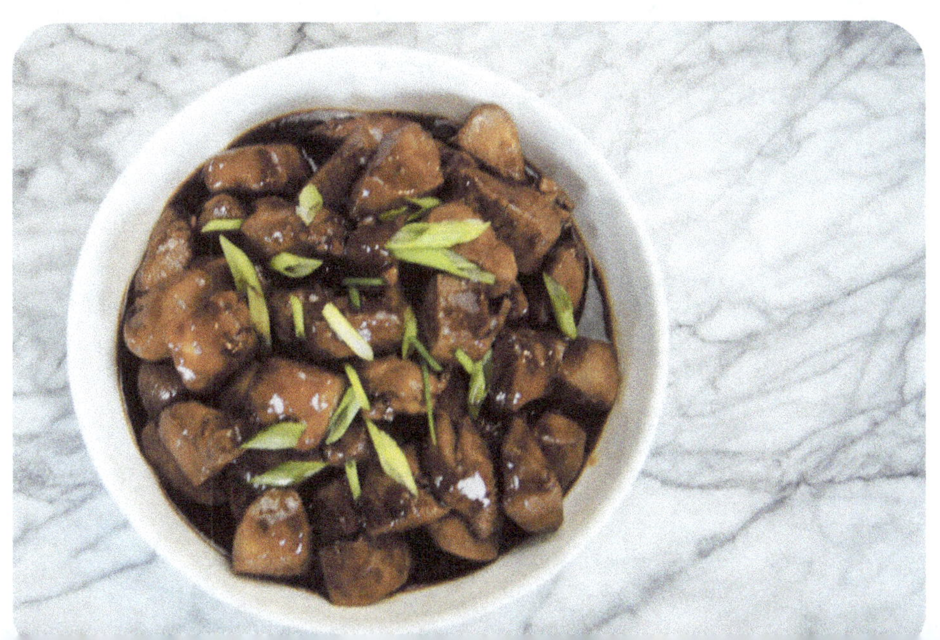

PROTEIN MEAT	**Tuna Cake** **Serves 4-6 patties**	**Main**
INGREDIENTS		**SUBSTITUTE**
2	5 oz cans of tuna	Canned salmon
¼ C	Mayonnaise	
2 Tbsp	Onion, finely diced	1 Tbsp dehydrated onion +1 Tbsp water
2 Tbsp	Red pepper, finely diced	Diced celery or olives or capers
1 tsp	Chili sauce (optional)	½ tsp red pepper flakes
1 Tbsp	Dijon mustard	½ Tbsp Worcestershire sauce
2	Eggs, large or XL	
¼ C	Bread crumbs, Panko	Any bread crumb or crushed cracker
2 Tbsp	Extra Virgin Olive Oil	Any olive oil light oil for pan frying
STEPS		
1	Drain tuna and break apart in a bowl.	
2	Mix in mayonnaise, onion, pepper, chili sauce, mustard and eggs.	
3	Add bread crumbs and mix gently. Mixture should hold together. Add more crumbs if needed.	
4	Form mixture into patties about ¾ inch thick. Makes about four large or six small patties. Chill patties briefly to help them hold their shape.	
5	Pan fry the patties in oil over medium high heat until golden brown and crispy – about four minutes per side.	
6	Serve alone or on a sandwich with a condiment such as mayo, dijonnaise, rémoulade, tartar sauce or a lemon wedge.	

PROTEIN MEAT	**Tuna Salad** **Serves 2-4**	**Main**
INGREDIENTS		**SUBSTITUTE**
2	5 oz cans of tuna	
2 Tbsp	Pickle relish, sweet	Diced dill pickle or olives or capers
2	Green onion, sliced	2 Tbsp red onion, diced
2	Ribs celery, diced	Red bell pepper, diced
½ C	Mayonnaise	
1 tsp	Dijon mustard (optional)	
STEPS		
1	Drain tuna well and break apart in a bowl.	
2	Add all remaining ingredients and mix well.	
3	Serve on bread, crackers, lettuce cups, tomato or cucumber slices or on salad greens.	
OPTIONS		
A	**Mediterranean**: Replace sweet pickle relish with capers or sliced olives. Replace celery with red pepper. Use 2-3 Tbsp diced red onion in place of green onion. Replace mayonnaise with 2 Tbsp Extra Virgin Olive Oil and 1 Tbsp lemon juice.	

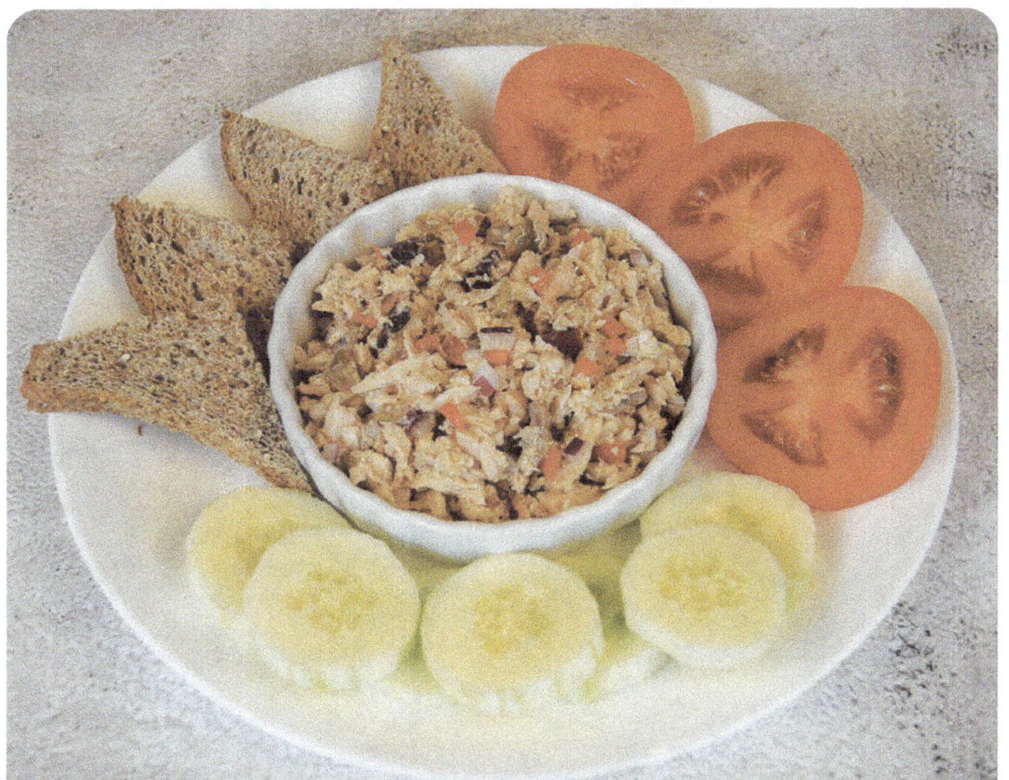

Mediterranean Tuna Salad

PROTEIN MEAT	**Yogurt Marinated Chicken** **Serves 4-6**	**Main**
INGREDIENTS		**SUBSTITUTE**
1-1½ lb	Chicken breast – whole, fillets or kabobs	Cut up chicken pieces or thighs (double weight if on the bone w/ skin)
1 C	Yogurt, plain Greek	Plain yogurt
1 Tbsp	Lemon juice	Lime juice or orange juice
2	Garlic cloves, minced	1 tsp minced jarred garlic
1 tsp	Paprika	
2 tsp	Cumin	
½ tsp	Oregano	1 tsp ginger paste
	Salt and pepper to taste	
STEPS		
1	Mix yogurt, lemon juice and spices together in a large Ziploc bag.	
2	Add chicken to the bag and turn to coat all surfaces.	
3	Press air from the bag, seal it and refrigerate for four hours to overnight.	
4	Remove chicken from the marinade and shake off any excess. Discard leftover marinade.	
5	Cook chicken over high heat. This can be on the grill, pan fried on the stove top, or roasted in a 400°F oven. Chicken is done when it reaches 165°F internal temperature.	
6	Goes well with any rice, bread, naan or pita.	
OPTIONS		
A	**Greek:** Omit the paprika and cumin, then double the amount of lemon, garlic and oregano.	
B	**Middle East Kabob:** Omit the paprika and cumin. Double the garlic and oregano, and add 2 tsp tomato paste, and ¼ tsp each cinnamon and allspice.	
C	**Tandoori:** Omit the oregano, reduce the cumin to 1 tsp and double the paprika. Add 1 tsp ginger paste, ½ tsp each cinnamon and coriander.	

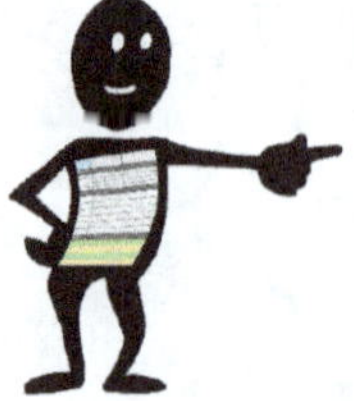

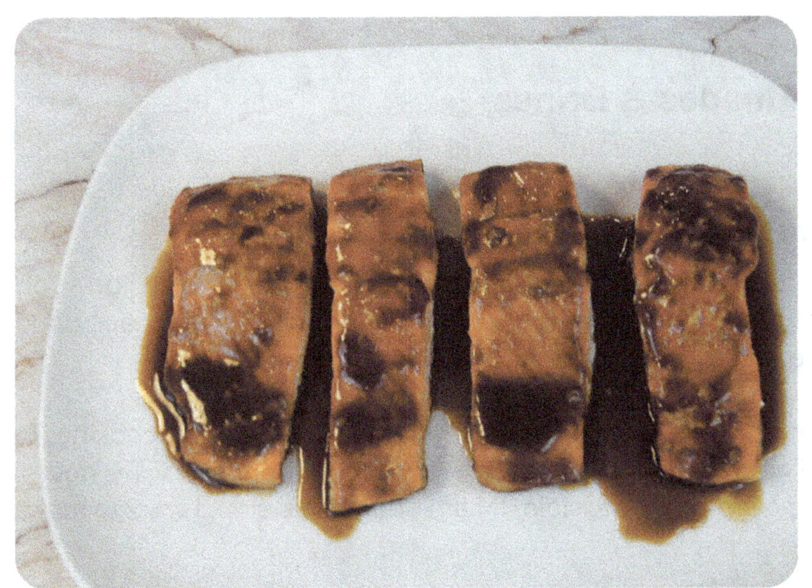

Glazed Salmon

Recipe on page 116

Shrimp Scampi

Recipe on page 118

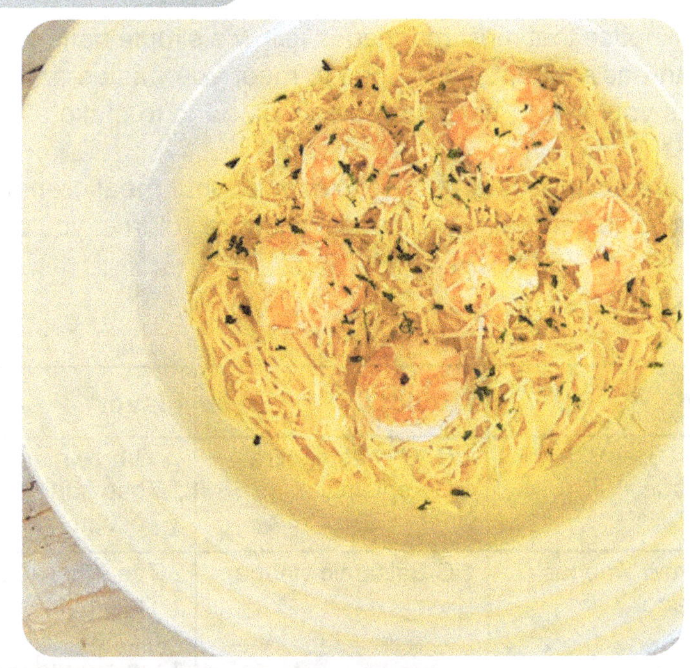

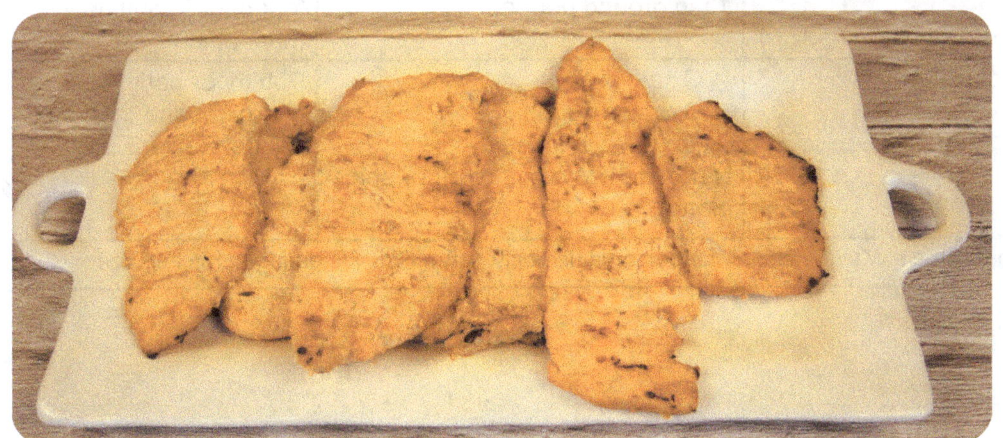

Yogurt Marinated

Chicken

Previous page

Marinades & Brines

Marinades and brines are great ways to create delicious meat dishes with minimum effort. You can always buy prepared marinades in the grocery store, but making your own is quick, easy and inexpensive. Additionally, you have more control over the ingredients and volume.

Marinades and brines often tenderize the meat and help keep it from drying out during cooking, in addition to imparting flavor. Thinly sliced meat and fish can get by with a quick marinate of 1-2 hours. However, I always prefer several hours to overnight if possible. If I am adding this step, I want to make it count!

You will notice that most marinades follow a simple pattern, making them ideal to put in a tabular form. You can easily adapt the recipes to meet your tastes and ingredients on hand. It is probably safe to say that you always have ingredients on hand to make a marinade.

Below are several easy recipes to expand your meat preparation repertoire. Each recipe is for about 3 lb of meat. In general, if you need a bit more volume, you can add an additional ¼- ½ C water or wine.

Type	Liquid	Flavor	For
Apple Cider Vinegar Marinade	1 C Worcestershire 1 C Apple cider vinegar	½ C brown sugar 1 Tbsp garlic, minced 1 Tbsp thyme or other herb	Pork tenderloin, loin roast, or pork chops
Balsamic Vinegar Marinade	1 C Balsamic vinegar	2 Tbsp brown sugar 1 Tbsp minced garlic 1 tsp salt 1 tsp ground pepper	For any steak, especially skirt or flank steak. Pierce meat with fork prior to putting in marinade.
Brown Sugar Brine	1 qt water	¼ C salt ½ C brown sugar 2 tsp garlic, minced Herbs de Provence or other spice blend	Poultry or pork. Soak overnight and then pat dry before cooking.

Type	Liquid	Flavor	For
Citrus Marinade	1 C orange juice ¼ C EVOO	1 Tbsp honey 1 tsp salt 2 tsp basil ½ tsp white pepper	Chicken (4-24 hours) or fish (2 hours)
Fajita Marinade	¼ C Orange Juice ¼ C Lime Juice ¼ C EVOO	1 tsp garlic, minced 2 tsp chili powder 1 tsp cumin 1 Tbsp cilantro (opt) 1 tsp salt	Marinate chicken or steak for 2-24 hours before grilling.
Greek Marinade	½ C EVOO ¼ C vinegar 2 Tbsp lemon juice	2 Tbsp garlic, minced 1 Tbsp sugar 2 tsp basil 2 tsp oregano 1 tsp rosemary 1 tsp salt ½ tsp black pepper ½ tsp red pepper flakes	Chicken or lamb. Great for kabobs. Marinade can be blended for a more intense flavor.
Italian Marinade	1 C EVOO ½ C vinegar (wine)	2 tsp salt 2 tsp garlic, minced 2 tsp oregano or Italian seasoning ½ tsp black pepper	Chicken, beef or lamb
Red Wine Marinade	1 C red wine ¼ C EVOO	2 tsp salt 2 Tsp rosemary 2 tsp garlic, minced 1 tsp black pepper ½ tsp red pepper flakes	Any steak, marinate over night
Teriyaki Marinade	½ C soy sauce ¼ C water 1 Tbsp vinegar (rice) 2 tsp sesame oil (opt)	1 Tbsp garlic, minced 1 Tbsp ginger, minced 4 Tbsp honey or sugar	Beef, pork, chicken, fish or tofu. Grill or pan fry, or use in stir fry.
Thyme Chicken Marinade	½ C EVOO 2 Tbsp lemon juice	2 Tbsp thyme (fresh) 1 Tbsp lemon zest 1 Tbsp parsley	Coat thin chicken cut-lets with paste. Rest for 4-24 hours.
Yogurt Marinade	1 C yogurt 1 Tbsp lemon juice	1 tsp salt 1 tsp garlic, minced 2 tsp cumin 1 tsp paprika ½ tsp oregano	Chicken, marinate for 6–24 hours.

VEGGIE	Bean Salad[V] Serves 8-10	Salad
INGREDIENTS		**SUBSTITUTE**
1	14.5 oz can, kidney beans	Black beans
1	14.5 oz can, white navy beans	Cannellini beans, black eyed peas
1	14.5 oz can, wax beans	
1	14.5 oz can, green beans	Fresh or frozen green beans, cooked
½	Onion, diced	
½	Bell pepper, diced, red or green	
1	Rib, celery, diced	
½ C	Canola oil	Any light, neutral oil
½ C	Apple cider vinegar	Any vinegar
¼ C	White sugar	
	Salt and pepper to taste	
STEPS		
1	Rinse and drain all of the canned beans.	
2	Whisk the oil, vinegar and sugar (or other dressing) together.	
3	Mix all ingredients. Cover and chill for several hours before serving.	
OPTIONS		
A	**Classic**: Recipe above with green bell peppers. Add ½ C chopped jarred pimento peppers if desired.	
B	**Southern**: Replace all of the beans with four cans of black eyed peas. Add 12 oz of cherry tomatoes, halved. Use 1 C of Dijon Vinaigrette dressing (page 140) instead of oil, vinegar and sugar.	
C	**Tex-Mex**: Use one can each of black beans and black eyed peas. Add 8 oz of halved cherry tomatoes and a 14.5 oz can corn (drained). Replace sugar with 1 tsp each chili powder and cumin.	
D	**Greek**: Replace green and wax beans with one can of chickpeas. Add 1 C diced cucumber and 8 oz halved cherry tomatoes. Use 1 C of the Greek salad dressing (page 141) in place of the oil, vinegar and sugar. Garnish with crumbled feta.	

VEGGIE	**Brussels Sprouts Salad**[V] **Serves 6-8**	**Salad**
INGREDIENTS		**SUBSTITUTE**
1½ lb	Brussels sprouts, fresh	
2	Apples	Pears
¾ C	Cherries, dried	Dried cranberries
¾ C	Almonds, sliced	Sunflower seeds, pumpkin seeds or toasted, chopped walnuts
¾ C	Parmesan cheese, grated	Sharp cheddar cheese
1 C	Honey Mustard Salad Dressing (page 141)	Lemon, Orange or Raspberry Vinaigrette dressing (page 141)
STEPS		
1	Cut Brussels sprouts into thin slices with knife or mandolin.	
2	Toss the Brussels sprouts with the dressing and allow to stand while preparing the other ingredients to allow the sprouts to soften.	
3	Peel apples if desired and then dice into small pieces. May be grated.	
4	Toss remaining ingredients with the Brussels sprouts and serve.	

For a change of pace, try purple Brussels sprouts:

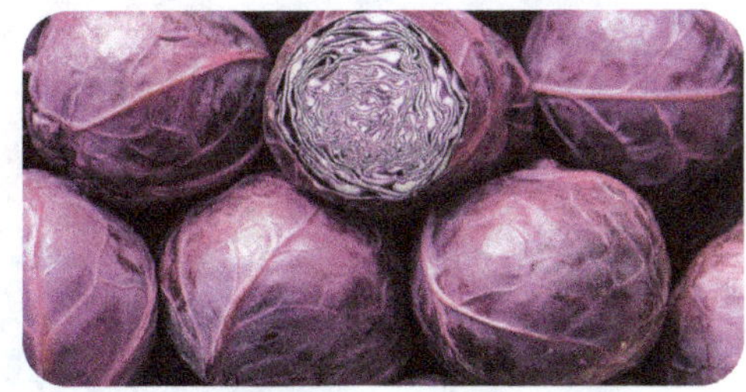

- **Typically harvested in the fall.**
- **Milder and sweeter flavor than green Brussels sprouts.**
- **Flavor and color makes them great in salads.**

VEGGIE	Carrot Salad w/ Fruit[V] Serves 4-6	Salad
INGREDIENTS		**SUBSTITUTE**
1 lb	Carrots, grated	Bagged grated or matchstick carrots
¾ C	Mayonnaise	Yogurt, plain or vanilla. Omit honey if using sweetened.
1 Tbsp	Lemon juice	Apple cider vinegar
2 Tbsp	Honey	
1	20 oz can crushed pineapple, drained	1 apple, diced
½ C	Raisins, separated	Dried cranberries or cherries
½ C	Pecans, chopped	Walnuts or ¼ C sunflower seeds
STEPS		
1	In a good size bowl, mix the mayonnaise, lemon juice and honey until smooth.	
2	Add remaining ingredients and toss until combined. Refrigerate until ready to serve.	

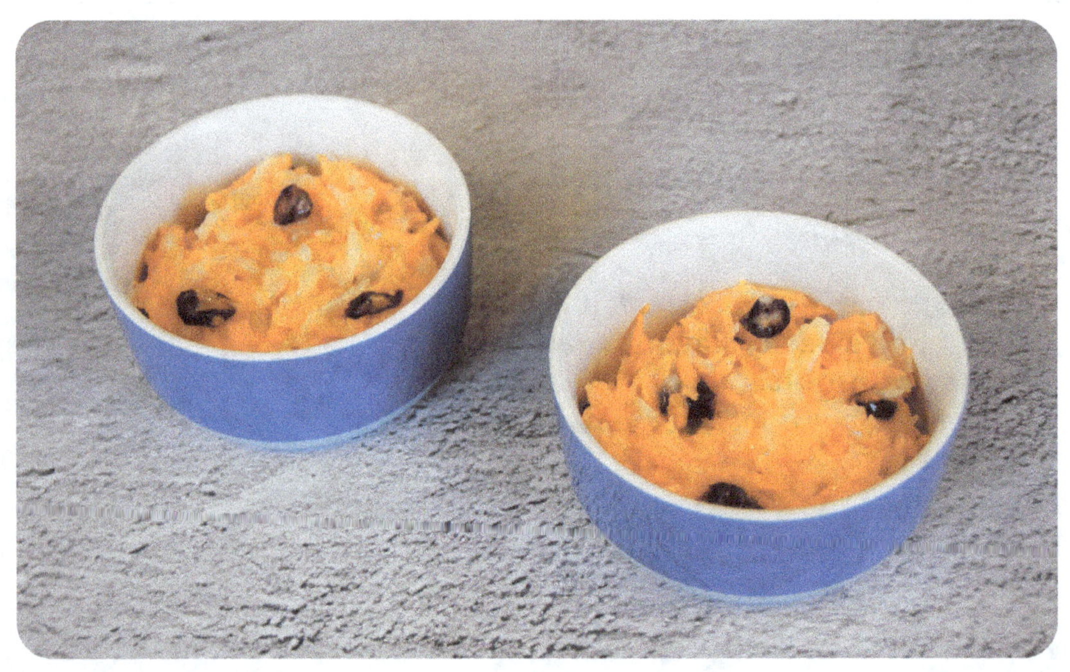

VEGGIE	Cucumber Salads[V] Serves 4-6	Salad
INGREDIENTS		**SUBSTITUTE**
2	Cucumbers, (about 2 pounds)	Hot house or English
½	Red onion, medium, sliced thinly	White, yellow or green onions
3 Tbsp	Dill, fresh	2 tsp dried dill, fresh basil or parsley
2 Tbsp	Extra Virgin Olive Oil	
½ C	Apple cider vinegar	Any vinegar, lemon juice
1 Tbsp	Sugar	
	Salt and pepper to taste	
STEPS		
1	Cucumbers may be peeled or not, depending on your preference. Slice cucumbers into disks.	
2	Mix all ingredients in a bowl, cover and chill.	
OPTIONS		
A	**Creamy:** Omit the sugar, oil and vinegar. Add ¼ C each of mayonnaise and sour cream (or Greek yogurt).	
B	**Greek:** Omit the sugar and apple cider vinegar. Replace the dill with 2 tsp oregano. Increase the Extra Virgin Olive Oil to ¼ C and add 2 Tbsp of lemon juice. Add 2 diced tomatoes, ½ C of black or Kalamata olives, and 4 oz Feta cheese.	

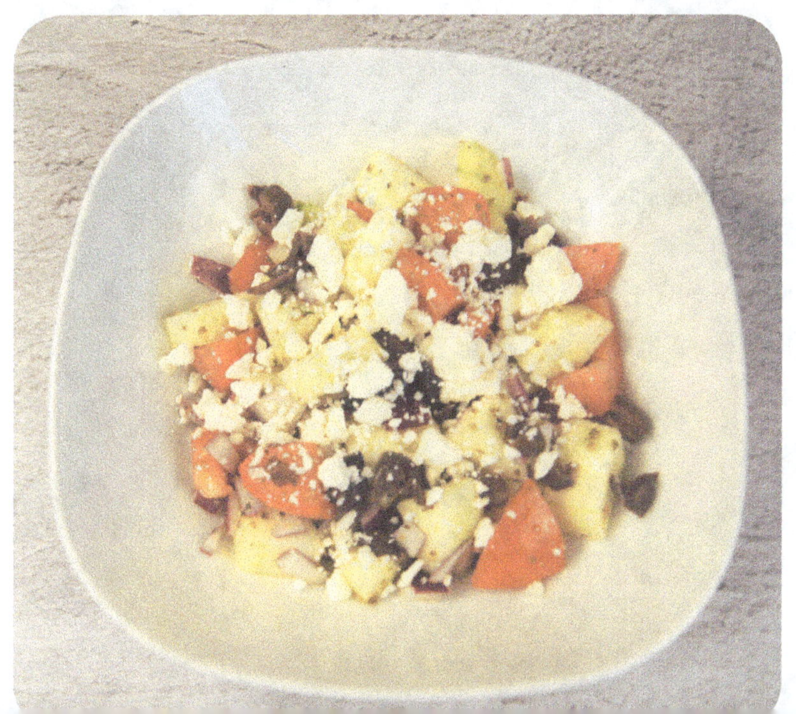

VEGGIE	**Green Bean Salad w/ Goat Cheese**[V] **Serves 4**	**Salad**
INGREDIENTS		**SUBSTITUTE**
2 lb	Fresh green beans	Frozen whole green beans
½ C	Orange Basil Vinaigrette (recipe page 141)	
4 oz	Goat cheese, crumbled	
½ C	Walnuts, chopped	Pecans
STEPS		
1	Steam green beans until they are tender crisp. Cool by putting them in ice water for five minutes or refrigerate for later use.	
2	Toss cool, drained green beans with the dressing.	
3	Garnish with crumbled goat cheese and chopped walnuts.	

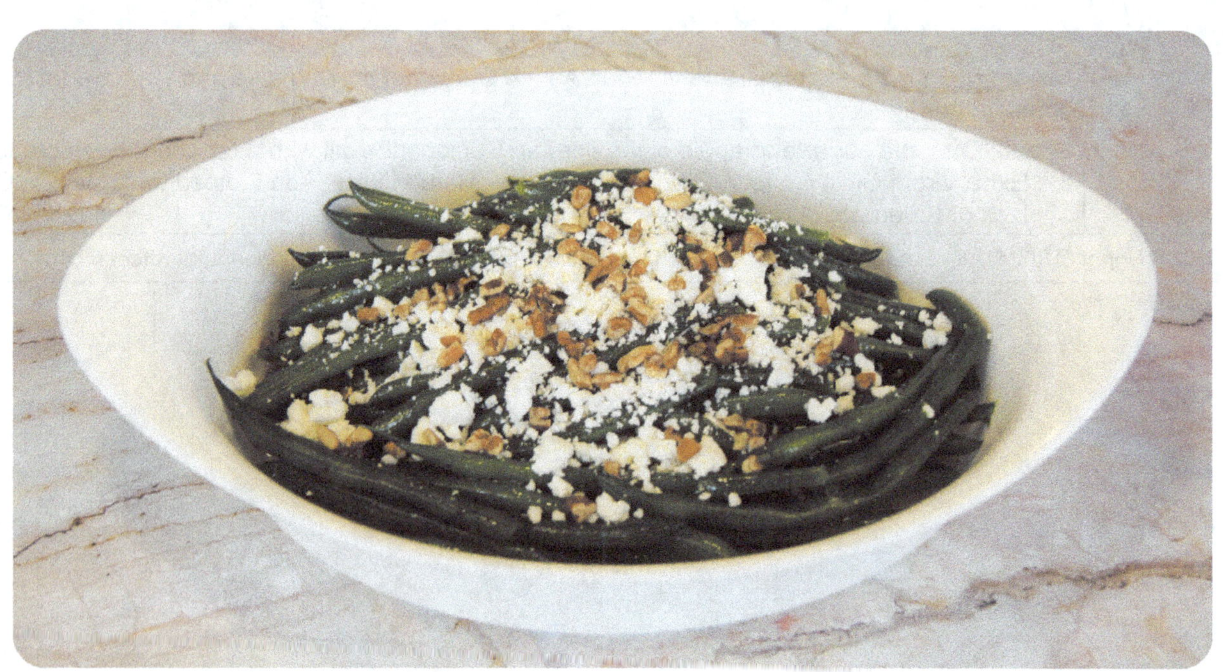

VEGGIE	Napa Cabbage Salad[V] Makes 6 side salads	Salad
INGREDIENTS		**SUBSTITUTE**
1	Head napa cabbage (large)	
2-3	Carrots, grated or julienned	
6	Green onions, finely sliced	
1	Orange, peeled and cut	Mandarin orange sections, drained
½	Red bell pepper, finely sliced (optional)	
½ C	Sliced almonds	Peanuts
~ ½ C	Ginger Soy Salad Dressing (recipe pg 140)	
STEPS		
1	Finely slice the cabbage.	
2	Combine all ingredients and toss.	
3	Serve plain or top with grilled chicken and crispy wantons.	

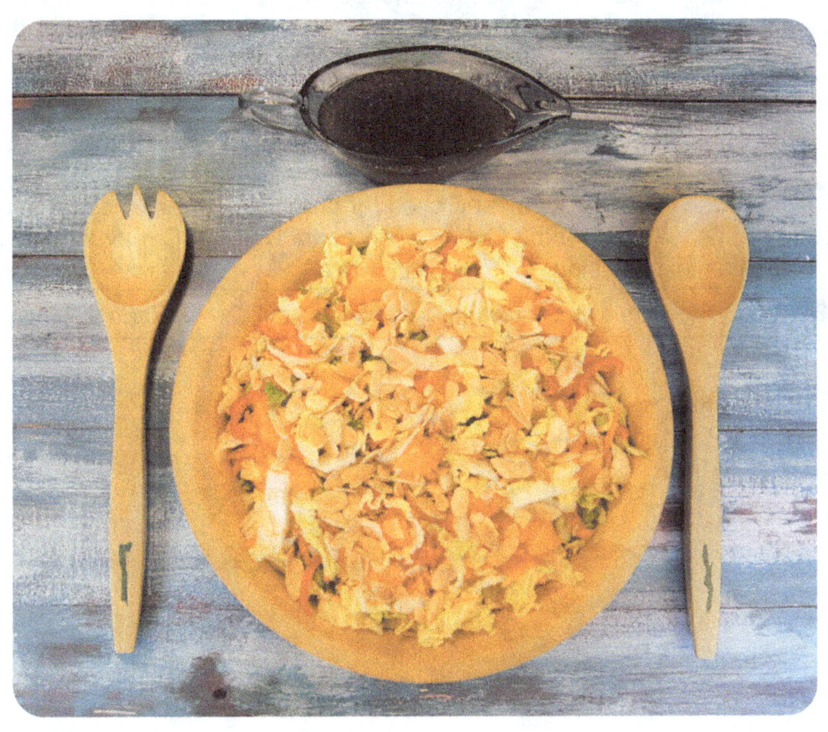

GRAIN	Pasta Salad[V] Serves 10-12	Salad
INGREDIENTS		**SUBSTITUTE**
1 lb	Pasta, any shape	
1	Onion, small, red, diced	Green, white or yellow onion
1	Red bell pepper, diced	Green pepper
1 pint	Tomatoes, cherry	
4 C	Broccoli, cut into bite sized florets	
8 oz	Cheddar cheese, grated	
1½ C	Ranch Salad Dressing (recipe on page 141)	Any salad dressing
STEPS		
1	Cook pasta to al dente then rinse in cold water and drain well.	
2	Steam the broccoli until tender but still crisp. Rinse in cold water and drain well.	
3	Toss all ingredients together, chill and serve.	
OPTIONS		
A	**Greek:** Omit the broccoli and cheddar cheese. Add 1 diced cucumber, 1 C Kalamata or black olives, and 8 oz crumbled feta cheese. Use Greek salad dressing instead of Ranch (shown on page 141).	
B	**Italian:** Omit the broccoli and cheddar cheese. Add 6 oz salami in small pieces, 1 C sliced black olives and 8 oz of shredded mozzarella. Use Lemon or Balsamic Vinaigrette dressing (pages 140 and 141).	
C	**Tuna:** Omit the tomato, broccoli and cheddar cheese. Add two 5 oz cans of tuna (drained), 3 diced hard boiled eggs and 2 C of cooked peas. Use 1½ C mayonnaise and ¼ C sweet pickle relish as the dressing.	

GRAIN	Rice Salad[V] Serves 8-10	Salad
INGREDIENTS		**SUBSTITUTE**
4 C	Rice, cooked al dente (1⅓ C uncooked)	White or brown
1	Red bell pepper, diced	
1	Red onion, small, diced	Green onion
2	Celery stalks, diced	
2	Carrots, diced	
½ - ¾ C	Lemon Vinaigrette (see recipe on page 141)	Any salad dressing
STEPS		
1	Rice should be cooked so that it is no longer crunchy but not mushy. Chill before using.	
2	Mix all ingredients and then chill prior to serving.	
OPTIONS		
A	**Mediterranean:** Omit the carrot and celery. Add one 15 oz can of white beans or chickpeas, ½ C Kalamata or black olives and ½ C feta cheese. Use Greek salad dressing shown on page 287.	
B	**Tex-Mex:** Omit the carrot and celery. Add one 15 oz can of black beans, one 15 oz can of corn, and two diced tomatoes. Dress with ½ C EVOO, ¼ C lime juice and ½ tsp each chili powder and cumin. Fresh cilantro and avocado are optional but nice additions.	

PROTEIN MEAT	Tuna Salad Niçoise Serves ~ 2	Salad
INGREDIENTS		**SUBSTITUTE**
1	Head of romaine	Any type of lettuce
2 C	Green beans, fresh (12-16 oz)	Frozen, whole
1	5 oz can of tuna (high quality)	
1	Potato, medium Russet, sliced	Any type of potato
1	Tomato, cut into wedges	
2	Eggs, hard boiled, quartered	
¼ C	Olives, Kalamata	Any type of olive
½ C	Dijon Vinaigrette Salad Dressing (page 140)	Lemon Vinaigrette, Greek or Caesar Dressings shown on pages 140 & 141
STEPS		
1	Steam green beans to tender crisp. Cool under cold water, drain well and chill.	
2	Cook potato by boiling until just tender but not mushy. Drain well and chill.	
3	Assemble salad: bed of greens, topped with remaining ingredients. Drizzle with dressing.	

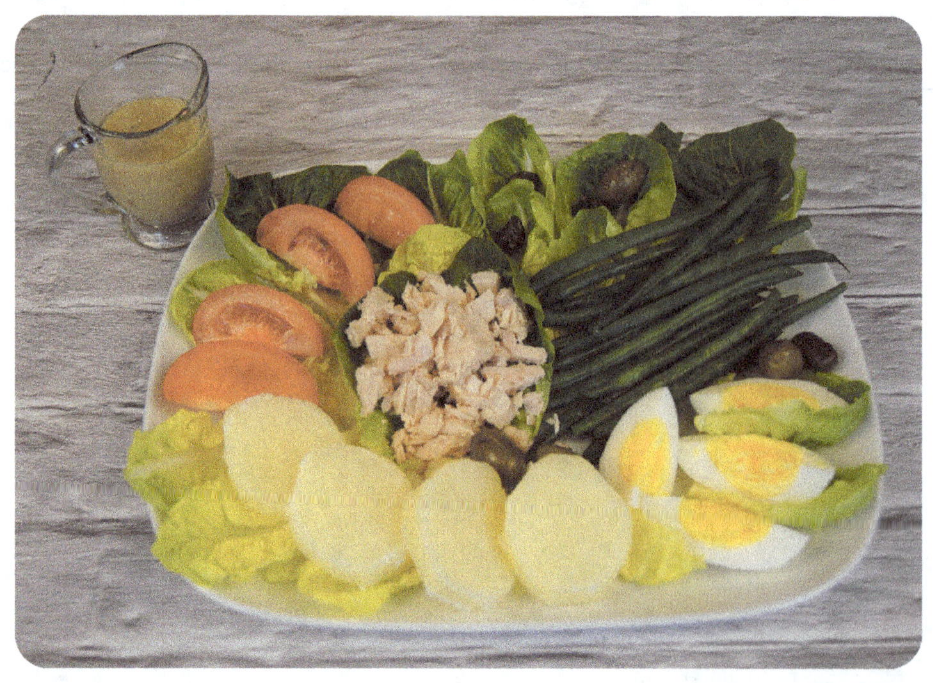

Salad Dressings

I like salads but I love salad dressings! There are many good, prepared salad dressings available in the grocery store. However, I no longer rely on them. This is an area where many people default to purchasing bottled dressings, assuming that making your own is complicated. It is not. On the following pages there are recipes for several common types of dressings. The creamy ones also serve well as dips. You should never feel that you can't make a salad because you are "out of dressing".

When you make your own dressing, you make the right volume and can control the ingredients. For example, you may choose to use high-quality olive oil and balsamic vinegar, avoiding seed oils, sugar, MSG, modified food starch, and preservatives. When you make your own dressing, you save money in two ways. ***The first way you save is by reducing waste.*** How many partial bottles of salad dressing have you discarded over the years? A certain percentage tends to be thrown out because it is hard to match use to the product size. On the other hand, staple ingredients like olive oil and vinegar are generally used completely. ***The second way you save is that home-made dressing costs less than one-half per ounce to make vs. pre-made dressings – even using high quality ingredients!***

Salad Dressing Tips & Tricks:

- » Multiply the recipes to get the desired volume.
- » To mellow the flavor of fresh garlic, microwave the oil and garlic for 15 seconds on high, then allow to cool.
- » A few drops of water added to vinaigrettes help emulsify the oil and vinegar. Not essential, but helpful if serving dressing on the side.
- » Can substitute garlic powder for crushed garlic.
- » Can substitute dehydrated onion flakes for grated onion.
- » Types of vinegar can be interchanged with minimal effect.
- » Extra Virgin Olive Oil can be replaced with canola or any light vegetable oil.
- » Plain or Greek yogurt can be substituted for sour cream.
- » If you have a little prepared non-creamy dressing left but need a bit more, add equal amounts of oil and vinegar to the bottle to get the desired volume. If it is a creamy dressing, add a little mayo, sour cream, or yogurt, thinned with milk. Shake well.
- » Fresh Buttermilk substitute – for ¼ C
  - » Prepared powdered buttermilk per package directions
  - » Mix ¼ C milk with 1 tsp lemon juice or vinegar and sit 10 minutes
  - » Mix 3 Tbls yogurt or sour cream with 1 Tbls milk

Simple Salad Dressings
Makes ~ ½ C, enough for 2 entree or 4 side salads

Type	Oil	Acid	Sweet	Flavoring
Balsamic Vinaigrette	¼ C EVOO	¼ C Balsamic vinegar	N/A	½ tsp garlic ¼ tsp pepper ½ tsp salt ½ tsp basil (or any herb)
Blue Cheese	¼ C mayo	¼ C sour cream	⅛ tsp sugar	1 Tbsp blue cheese crumbles ⅛ tsp pepper 1 Tbsp milk
Caesar	⅓ C mayo 1 tsp EVOO	1 Tbsp lemon juice	N/A	½ tsp garlic ¼ tsp Dijon mustard 1 tsp Worcestershire 1 Tbsp grated Parmesan
Coleslaw - Classic	¼ C mayo	¼ C apple cider vinegar	1 tsp sugar	¼ tsp salt ¼ tsp pepper ¼ tsp celery seed (opt)
Coleslaw - Russian	¼ C mayo	¼ C sour cream	⅛ tsp sugar	1 Tbsp grated onion
Creamy Dill	¼ C mayo	¼ C sour cream	⅛ tsp sugar	1 tsp dill ⅛ tsp pepper ¼ tsp salt 1 Tbsp milk
Dijon Vinaigrette	6 Tbsp EVOO	2 Tbsp vinegar	N/A	2 tsp Dijon mustard ½ tsp dehydrated onion ½ tsp salt ¼ tsp pepper
French	⅓ C EVOO	1½ Tbsp wine vinegar	¾ tsp sugar	½ tsp garlic 1½Tbsp chili sauce 1 tsp Worcestershire
Ginger Soy	¼ C EVOO	2 Tbsp rice vinegar	1 Tbsp honey	1 tsp ginger paste 1 Tbsp soy sauce ½ tsp garlic

Simple Salad Dressings
Makes ~ ½ C, enough for 2 entree or 4 side salads

Type	Oil	Acid	Sweet	Flavoring
Greek	¼ C EVOO	¼ C wine vinegar	N/A	½ tsp garlic ¼ tsp Dijon mustard ¼ tsp oregano ¼ tsp basil ¼ tsp pepper ¼ tsp salt ¼ tsp onion powder Feta cheese on salad
Honey Mustard	¼ C EVOO	3 Tbsp apple cider vinegar	2 Tbsp honey	2 Tbsp Dijon mustard
Lemon Vinaigrette	¼ C EVOO	2 Tbsp lemon juice 2 Tbsp white wine vinegar	1 tsp honey	½ tsp oregano ¼ tsp pepper ¼ tsp salt ¼ tsp dehydrated onion (opt)
Orange Basil Vinaigrette	¼ C EVOO	1 Tbsp orange juice concentrate 3 Tbsp white vinegar	1 tsp honey	1 tsp basil ¼ tsp pepper ¼ tsp salt
Ranch	¼ C mayo	¼ C buttermilk 1 Tbsp sour cream (opt)	N/A	1 tsp parsley ½ tsp dill ¼ tsp dehydrated onion ⅛ tsp garlic powder ⅛ tsp onion powder ⅛ tsp pepper ¼ tsp salt
Raspberry Vinaigrette	¼ C EVOO	¼ C raspberry vinegar	1 Tbsp raspberry preserves	¼ tsp basil ⅛ tsp pepper ¼ tsp salt
Sweet Vinegar	¼ C EVOO	⅓ C apple cider vinegar	3 Tbsp sugar	½ tsp salt
Thousand Island	½ C mayo	N/A	1 tsp sweet pickle relish	1 tsp ketchup 1 tsp minced onion, fresh or dehydrated

Sauces

Sometimes even a simple little sauce can take a dish from "meh" to "mmm". Recipes for making lovely dishes with intricate sauces are readily available so we don't need to talk about them here. If you are making Veal Piccata or Eggs Benedict with scratch-made Hollandaise to impress the in-laws, the internet has you covered. What we include here are a few of the most basic, easy sauces and then some even easier short-cut sauces. These sauces exist for moments when you are thinking, "Gee, a little sauce would really help."

The line between sauce and gravy is only flavor, not technique. If it tastes like meat, we tend to call it gravy. For our purposes, a sauce is any thickened liquid that adds flavor, whether it be sweet or savory. The most common sauces use either flour or corn starch as a thickening agent, so we have included recipes for a basic Flour-Roux Sauce and a Corn Starch Sauce, each with several variations. There are also recipes for several cooking sauces that are commonly purchased. And then we have the short-cut sauces that are so quick and easy that it almost feels like cheating. These short-cut sauces may not win any culinary awards, but when you've conjured a sauce out of almost nothing, it seems like magic.

Sauce Type	Ingredients	Method
Caramel	2 Tbsp butter 2 Tbsp brown sugar 1 tsp milk or cream	Mix in microwave safe bowl. Microwave on 60% power in 15 second increments, stirring in between, until melted and fairly smooth (not perfect). Serve with ice cream or other desserts.
Cocktail	¼ C ketchup 1 tsp prepared horseradish 1 tsp Worcestershire sauce ½ tsp lemon juice	Mix all ingredients and serve with shrimp.
Dijonnaise	2 Tbsp mayo 1 tsp Dijon mustard	Mix. Use to jazz up your sandwiches or salads.
Fondue Cheat	1 C white wine 1 Tbsp corn starch 2 C grated cheese (mix of types)	Mix cold wine and corn starch in a small pan. Warm over very low heat until thickened. Mix in cheese and stir until melted. Serve as dip, can keep warm in a mini crock pot.
Fruit Dip	1 C Greek yogurt, plain 8 oz cream cheese 1/4 C honey, maple syrup, or fruit preserves 1 tsp vanilla extract	Combine all ingredients in a bowl and beat until smooth. Serve as a dip with fresh fruit or as a creamy topping for any dessert.

Sauce Type	Ingredients	Method
Fruit Sauce/Glaze	½ C fruit juice (any flavor) ½ Tbsp corn starch 2 Tbsp jam or preserves	Mix cold juice and corn starch in a small pan. Warm over low heat, stirring until thickened. Stir in jam or preserves until smooth. Serve as a glaze or sauce for meat or poultry, or as a topping for desserts, pancakes etc.
Instant Marinara	1 C tomato sauce 1 tsp oregano 1 tsp onion powder ½ tsp garlic powder ½ tsp basil ¼ tsp red pepper flakes (opt)	Mix together and warm. Use as a pizza sauce, dipping sauce, or to extend volume of any tomato-based sauce in cooking. Use to top vegetables, pasta or meat and then bake with cheese.
Magic Cheese	2 Tbsp sour cream 2 Tbls milk or cream 2 oz grated cheese Salt and pepper to taste	Mix in microwave safe bowl. Microwave on 60% power in 15 second increments, stirring in between, until melted and smooth. Serve with veggies, pasta, rice, potatoes, etc.
Mayonnaise 1	1 large egg (pasteurized) ¾ C canola oil 1 Tbsp lemon juice or vinegar 1 tsp salt ¼ tsp pepper 1 tsp Dijon mustard (opt)	Mix all ingredients except oil. Add oil gradually, and whip until emulsified using whisk, immersion blender, blender or food processor
Mayonnaise 2	1 hard boiled egg – XL ¼ C canola oil 1 tsp lemon juice ¼ tsp salt 1 tsp Dijon mustard	Mix all ingredients and blend for several minutes until emulsified and creamy using immersion blender, blender or food processor.
Orange Honey Ginger Syrup	½ C water ½ C white sugar 2 Tbsp OJ concentrate 2 Tbsp honey 2 tsp ginger paste or crystallized ginger (minced)	Mix ingredients in a small saucepan and bring to a boil. Allow it to boil until it starts to thicken slightly then cool. Serve over fruit, desserts, pancakes or in drinks. Use as a glaze for chicken or fish.
Remoulade	½ C mayo 1 Tbsp Dijon or brown mustard 1 tsp lemon juice 1 tsp garlic powder ½ tsp paprika 1 tsp hot sauce 1 Tbsp ketchup 1 tsp chopped capers (opt)	Mix ingredients. Better if allowed to rest to meld flavors. Serve with fish, fries, chicken tenders, shrimp, asparagus or as a spread on a sandwich.

VEGGIE	Classic Marinara^V Makes about 2 cups	Sauce
INGREDIENTS		**SUBSTITUTE**
28 oz	One can whole tomatoes, high quality	Crushed or diced tomatoes
4 Tbsp	Extra Virgin Olive Oil	
½	Medium onion, finely diced	
8	Cloves fresh garlic, minced	4 tsp jarred minced garlic
½ tsp	Salt	
1 tsp	Basil	Oregano
⅛ tsp	Red pepper flakes (optional)	
STEPS		
1	Put tomatoes in a large bowl and crush into small pieces. May use hands but a pastry cutter or large fork work also.	
2	In a large, heavy bottomed pot, sauté the onion over medium heat until very soft – about five minutes.	
3	Add the garlic and continue cooking for another 1-2 minutes.	
4	Add all of the other ingredients to the pot. Bring to a boil and then reduce heat to simmer.	
5	Simmer uncovered for at least 20 minutes, stirring often. Sauce will thicken as it cooks.	
6	Serve over pasta or use in any recipe calling for a marinara-type sauce.	

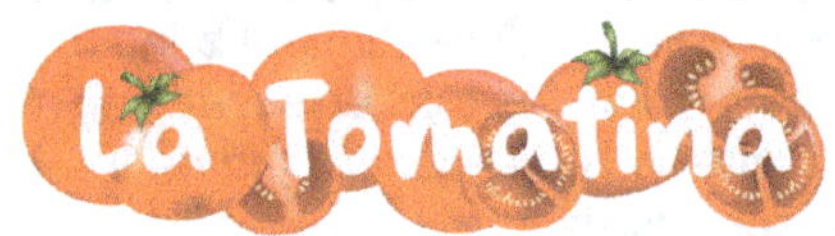

Bunol, Spain hosts the craziest tomato festival in the world each August. It is called La Tomatina and is said to be the world's largest food fight. About 20,000 participants pay to throw about 150,000 tomatoes at each other. In the end, they look like they are all swimming in Marinara sauce!

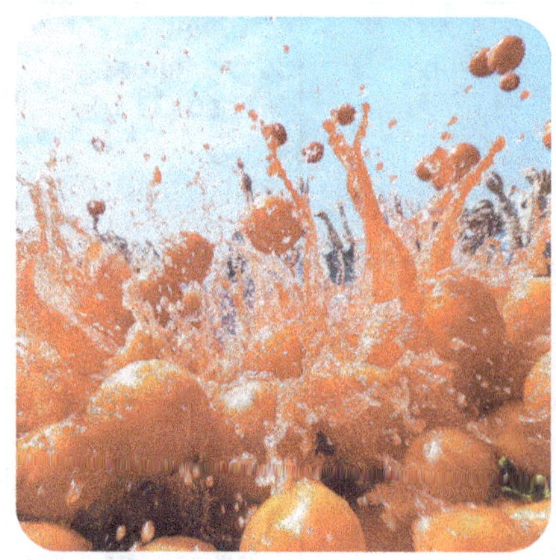

GRAIN	Corn Starch Sauces[V] Makes 1 cup	Sauce
INGREDIENTS		**SUBSTITUTE**
1 Tbsp	Corn starch	
1 C	Water, broth, juice, or wine - cool	Any clear liquid
	Liquid flavoring: include in liquid measure	Worcestershire, soy sauce, chili sauce, vinegar, lemon juice
	Seasoning additions	Salt, pepper, spices
STEPS		
1	Measure cold liquid including any liquid flavoring. Stir in corn starch until well mixed.	
2	Warm the corn starch and liquid mixture over medium heat, stirring until thickened. The cold corn starch mixture may be added directly to a pan with cooked food (e.g. stir fry) and warmed together as sauce thickens.	
3	Add seasoning and flavor additions to sauce. Return to heat only as necessary to fully incorporate and/or to warm.	
OPTIONS		
A	**Lemon Sauce**: Include 2 Tbsp of lemon juice in liquid. Dissolve ¼ C sugar in liquid before heating. Add grated lemon zest at the end. Serve as a topping for spice cake, pancakes or desserts.	
B	**Stir Fry**: Use ½ C each of water and soy sauce for the liquid. Add 2 tsp each ginger, garlic and sugar (or honey). Add 1 tsp chili sauce if desired. Mix well and add to pan with stir fry meat and/or veggies, stirring until thickened.	
C	**Mushroom Sauce**: Use wine or broth for liquid. Add 8-16 oz sauteéd mushrooms to thickened sauce. Add salt, pepper, garlic and herbs if desired.	
D	**Fruit Compote**: Use fruit juice for liquid (may be drained from canned or frozen fruit or other juce). Add ¼ - ½ C sugar to thickened sauce if needed. Stir in drained fruit and warm thoroughly.	

VEGGIE	Enchilada Sauce[V] Makes about 2½ cups		Sauce
INGREDIENTS		**SUBSTITUTE**	
1½ Tbsp	Extra Virgin Olive Oil	Any olive oil, cooking oil, or butter	
1 Tbsp	Flour		
1 C	Chicken stock	Beef or vegetable stock, or water	
1 Tbsp	Onion powder or dehydrated onion	½ C diced onion, sautéed	
½ tsp	Garlic powder or granules	1 tsp minced garlic	
1	Can (15 oz) tomato sauce	Diced, crushed or pureed canned tomatos, blended	
1½ Tbsp	Chili powder		
1 Tbsp	Oregano		
½ Tbsp	Cumin		
1 Tbsp	Lemon juice		
½ tsp	Rosemary, ground		
¼ tsp	Pepper		
¼ tsp	Cayenne pepper (optional)		
STEPS			
1	In a medium suace pan, cook oil and flour over medium heat stirring often. Allow to bubble for for two to three minutes to make a light roux.		
2	Add stock to the roux and mix well. Cook over medium heat, stirring constantly to slightly thicken the stock mixture.		
3	Add all other ingredients to the sauce pan and simmer for at least 10 minutes (20 is better), stirring occasionally.		

GRAIN	Flour-Based Sauces[V] Makes about 1 cup	Sauce
INGREDIENTS		**SUBSTITUTE**
1½ Tbsp	Butter	Any oil or rendered meat fat.
1 Tbsp	Flour	
1 C	Milk	Broth, wine or other liquid compatible with flavors.
	Salt and pepper to taste	
STEPS		
1	Melt butter in small pan. Add flour.	
2	Cook flour and butter over medium low heat for at least three minutes. Should gently bubble. Flour and oil mixture (roux) may cook longer and will develop a nutty flavor as it browns.	
3	Remove pan from heat to cool slightly. Add all of the liquid, stirring to fully incorporate.	
4	Return pan to medium low heat, stirring constantly until the sauce thickens. Do not allow to come to a boil. Remove from heat when thickened.	
5	Add seasonings and additions to the sauce. Return to low heat only as necessary to fully incorporate and warm.	
OPTIONS		
A	**White Sauce**: Cook flour in butter for minimum time, use milk and then season with salt and ⅛ tsp nutmeg. Mix with any cooked veggie for creamed peas, red cabbage, corn, etc.	
B	**Cheese Sauce**: Use butter and milk. Stir in 2 C of grated cheese until melted. Add a little milk if sauce is too thick. A mixture of sharp and mild cheeses develop the best flavor. Season with salt, pepper, paprika. Serve over veggies like brocolli or 8 oz cooked pasta.	
C	**Roast Meat Gravy**: Use oil from pan drippings (just fat, no liquid!). Use strained, skimmed pan drippings and/or broth for the liquid. Salt and pepper to taste.	
D	**Mushroom Sauce**: Use any oil and milk, broth or wine to make the basic sauce. Stir in 8-16 oz mushrooms, sauteed with garlic. Season with salt, pepper, and basil. Serve with meat, poutry, eggs, potatoes or veggies.	
E	**Onion Gravy**: Use any oil and either milk or broth. Stir in 1 sliced onion which has been sauteéd to at least soft, preferably carmelized. Salt and pepper to taste. Great with pork.	

PROTEIN OTHER	**Gorganzola Cream Sauce**[V] **Makes 3 cups**	**Sauce**
INGREDIENTS		**SUBSTITUTE**
2 C	Heavy cream	
2 oz	Gorgonzola cheese, crumbled	Blue cheese
2 Tbsp	Parmesan cheese, grated	
2 Tbsp	Parsley, fresh chopped	1 Tbsp dry parsley or basil
	Salt and pepper to taste	
STEPS		
1	In a medium sauce pan, bring cream to a boil over medium heat.	
2	Continue to boil for 30-45 minutes, stirring occasionally. Boil until the volume has reduced by half and the cream has thickened.	
3	Remove from heat, add the remaining ingredients, and stir until smooth. Return to low heat if necessary to melt cheese.	
4	Serve this rich and full flavored sauce sparingly over pasta or veggies. Compliments squash, sweet potato, or pumpkin pastas exceptionally well.	

VEGGIE	Mushroom Parmesan Cream Sauce[V] Makes 3 cups	Sauce
INGREDIENTS		**SUBSTITUTE**
1-2 lb	Mushrooms, sliced (white or brown)	Any type or mix of mushrooms, frozen
2 Tbsp	Extra Virgin Olive Oil	
4	Cloves garlic	2 tsp minced jarred garlic
2 tsp	Basil	Parsley
¾ C	Heavy cream	¾ C milk blended with 1½ tsp flour
½ C	Parmesan cheese, grated	
½ tsp	Black pepper	
STEPS		
1	In a large sauté pan, cook the mushrooms and garlic in the oil until all of the moisture from the mushrooms has evaporated.	
2	Stir the basil and the heavy cream into the mushrooms, mixing well over low heat until it starts to thicken.	
3	Stir in the Parmesan cheese and pepper. Turn off heat and stir gently. The sauce should continue to thicken.	
4	Serve tossed with pasta or as a topping for grilled chicken, bruschetta, polenta or vegetables.	

VEGGIE	Spanish Sauce^V Makes about 2 cups	Sauce
INGREDIENTS		**SUBSTITUTE**
2 Tbsp	Extra Virgin Olive Oil	
2	Onions, medium, finely diced	
1	Green pepper, diced	Red bell pepper - sweeter taste
1½ tsp	Garlic, minced	
16 oz	Can, diced toimatoes	Tomato puree or whole, fresh tomatoes cut up
2 tsp	Paprika, sweet	Smoked paprika
	Salt and pepper to taste	
STEPS		
1	In a heavy sauce pan, sauté onion and pepper in the oil over medium heat until soft.	
2	Add minced garlic and continue cooking for an additional two minutes.	
3	Add tomatoes and paprika. Allow to simmer over medium-low heat until thickened, about 20 minutes.	
4	Optional Step: Blend with an immersion blender if you want a smooth sauce.	
5	Serve over eggs, grilled chicken or fish, rice, mild veggies like zucchini or cauliflower.	

TEMPERATURE

FAHRENHEIT	CELSIUS
100 °F	37 °C
150 °F	65 °C
200 °F	93 °C
250 °F	121 °C
300 °F	150 °C
325 °F	160 °C
350 °F	180 °C
375 °F	190 °C
400 °F	200 °C
425 °F	220 °C
450 °F	230 °C
500 °F	260 °C
525 °F	274 °C
550 °F	288 °C

GRAIN	$100 Macaroni & Cheese[V] Serves 8-10	Side
INGREDIENTS		**SUBSTITUTE**
1 lb	Pasta, penne or spirals	Any shape that does not pack tightly
3 Tbsp	Flour	
3 Tbsp	Butter	Extra Virgin Olive Oil
3 C	Milk	
6 oz	Sharp cheddar cheese	
6 oz	Swiss cheese (preferably aged)	
4 oz	Asiago or Parmesan cheese	
4 oz	Colby or Co-Jack cheese	
½ tsp	Salt	
STEPS		
1	Preheat oven to 350°F. Prepare a 9" x13" pan or 2½ quart baking dish by coating with cooking spray.	
2	Grate all of the cheese and mix together in a bowl. Measure cheese, including pre-shredded cheese, by weight.	
3	Cook the pasta to slightly less done than al dente and drain. It will cook more in the oven later.	
4	In a heavy bottomed sauce pan, melt butter and mix in the flour. Cook over medium heat for three to five minutes to cook flour.	
5	Remove from heat and add the milk. Stir to fully incorporate and then return to heat.	
6	Heat milk/flour mixture over medium heat, stirring constantly. Sauce will thicken as it comes to almost a boil. Turn off the heat.	
7	Stir in ¾ of the cheese to the sauce, reserving the remainder for topping. Allow the cheese to melt, only adding enough heat as is necessary to get a smooth sauce.	
8	Mix the pasta and sauce together, then pour in the prepared pan. Top with the remining grated cheese.	
9	Bake for 30-45 minutes, until bubbly and golden brown on top.	

Photo on page 169

VEGGIE	Aloo Gobi[V] Serves 6-8	Side
INGREDIENTS		**SUBSTITUTE**
1	Head cauliflower (about 2 lb)	
2-3	Potatoes (about 1½ lb)	
1 Tbsp	Ginger paste or grated ginger	
4	Cloves garlic	2 tsp minced garlic
2 Tbsp	Extra Virgin Olive Oil	Coconut oil, any olive or light oil
3 Tbsp	Curry powder or curry paste	1½ Tbsp coriander + 2 tsp cumin + ½ tsp turmeric + 2 tsp Garam Masala
½ tsp	Kashmiri chili powder (optional)	½ tsp red pepper flakes (optional)
1 C	Water	
1 tsp	Salt	
STEPS		
1	Cut cauliflower into one inch florets. Dice potatoes into similar size cubes.	
2	In a large pot with a lid, heat oil and add ginger and garlic. Cook for 1-2 minutes. Add spices and cook for another minute.	
3	Add potatoes, water and spices to the pot, stirring to coat potatoes. Put on the lid and cook over medium heat for about 10 minutes, stirring occasionally.	
4	Add the cauliflower and stir to coat pieces. Replace lid and cook for another 12-15 minutes, stirring occasionally, until cauliflower and potatoes are tender. Adjust the salt.	
5	Serve with rice or naan, and a garnish of cilantro leaves if desired.	

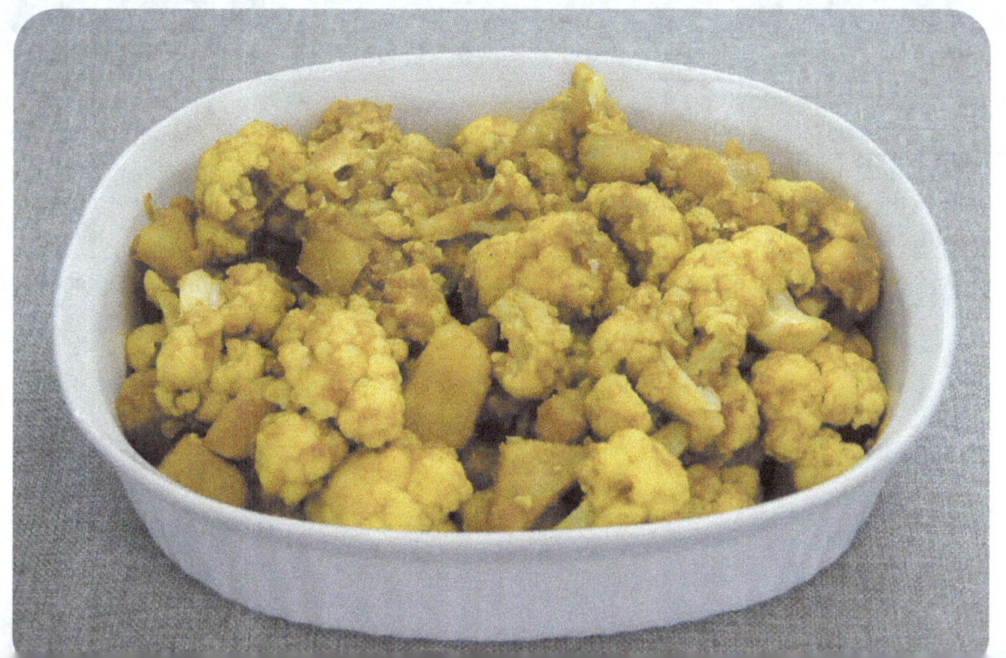

PROTEIN OTHER	**Beans & Rice**^{V} **Serves 4-6**	**Side**
INGREDIENTS		**SUBSTITUTE**
1 Tbsp	Extra Virgin Olive Oil	
1	Onion, diced	
½	Red or green bell pepper, diced	
2	Cloves garlic, minced	1 tsp jarred minced garlic
1 C	White rice, uncooked	
1	15.5 oz can red kidney beans, drained	Black beans
1	14.5 oz can diced tomatoes	
12 oz	Andouille sausage, diced	Smoked sausage, bacon
1 C	Chicken or vegetable stock	1 C water + 1 tsp stock paste
2 tsp	Cajun spice blend	
STEPS		
1	In a large pot with a lid, sauté the onion and pepper in the oil until it is soft. Add the garlic and cook for another minute.	
2	Stir sausage and spices in and cook over medium high heat for 3-4 minutes, stirring.	
3	Add tomatoes, rice, beans and stock and bring to a boil. Reduce heat to a simmer and cover pot.	
4	Simmer for 20 minutes with the lid in place and then stir. If rice is not yet done, return to heat for another five minutes.	
5	Remove from heat and allow to rest for five minutes with lid on. Salt to taste.	
OPTIONS		
A	**Dirty Rice**: Recipe above. Pairs well with fried okra, collard greens or cornbread.	
B	**Spanish Rice**: Omit the Andouille sausage. Replace the Cajun spice blend with 1 tsp paprika and ½ tsp each of cumin and oregano. Garnish with ¼ C sliced green olives.	
C	**Cuban Moro**: Replace sausage with four slices crumbled cooked bacon. Use black beans, omit the tomatoes, and add 1 C of water. Replace Cajun spice mix with ½ tsp each of cumin and oregano.	

Photo with Picadillo on page 113

VEGGIE	**Braised Cabbage**[V] **Makes ~ 8 cups**	**Side**
INGREDIENTS		**SUBSTITUTE**
1	Cabbage head, ~ 3 lb, cut into ½ inch slices	Red or green cabbage
1	Onion, medium sliced	Any type
3 - 5	Carrots, cut to ½ inch thick (optional)	
2 tsp	Stock paste, chicken	Bouillon powder or cubes, beef or vegetable
½ C	Water	
½ tsp	Salt and pepper, each	
1 Tbsp	Balsamic vinegar	1 Tbsp vinegar + 2 tsp sugar
2-3 Tbsp	Butter	
STEPS		
1	Layer cabbage, onion and carrots in the bottom of a large pot with a tight lid.	
2	Add water, stock paste, salt and pepper, then close lid.	
3	Cook over medium high heat for 10-15 minutes, stirring occasionally, until veggies are tender-crisp. Add a small amount of water only if necessary to keep pot from drying out.	
4	Stir in vinegar and butter. Cook uncovered for a few minutes, continuing to stir, until moisture is nearly gone.	
5	Serve plain or with a garnish of bread crumbs or bacon crumbles. Pairs nicely with cured or uncured pork, or sausage.	

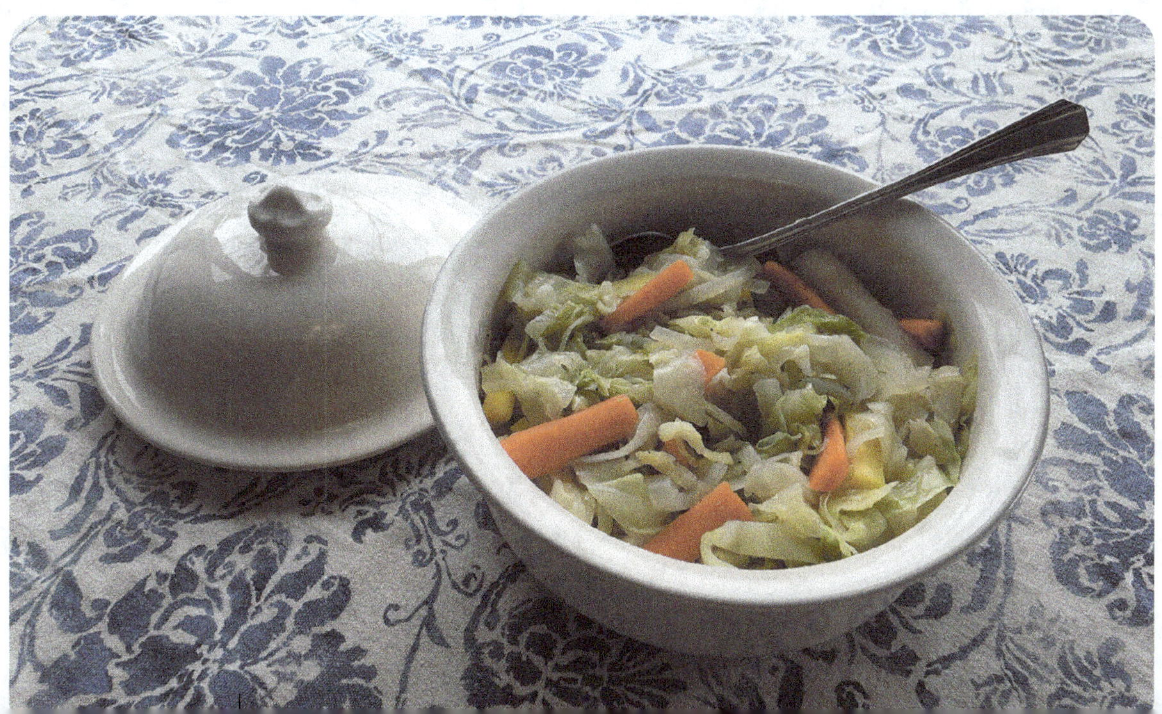

VEGGIE	Cauliflower & Sweet Potato Curry^{V} Serves 4-6	Side
INGREDIENTS		**SUBSTITUTE**
2 Tbsp	Extra Virgin Olive Oil	
1	Medium onion, sliced	
1 Tbsp	Curry paste	Curry powder
2 tsp	Garam Masala	
2	Medium sweet potatoes, diced	
1	15 oz can chopped tomatoes	Tomato sauce or 2 medium fresh tomatoes
½ C	Broth or stock	Water
1	Head cauliflower, cut into florets	
1	15 oz can chickpeas, rinsed and drained	
½ C	Heavy cream (optional)	Yogurt
STEPS		
1	In a large heavy bottomed pot, sauté the sliced onions in the olive oil over medium heat until translucent.	
2	Add the spices and diced sweet potatoes and continue to cook for 3 minutes while stirring.	
3	Add the tomatoes and broth to the pan and bring to a low boil. Cook for 10-15 minutes, until the sweet potatoes can be pierced with a fork.	
4	Add the chickpeas and the cauliflower florets to the pan and stir to combine. If it seems too dry, add an additional ½ C of broth or water.	
5	Place the lid on and allow to cook until the cauliflower is done to your preference - about 5-10 minutes. Stir occasionally.	
6	For a creamier result, stir the heavy cream or yogurt into the sauce.	
7	Serve alone or with rice, plain lentils, paratha or naan.	

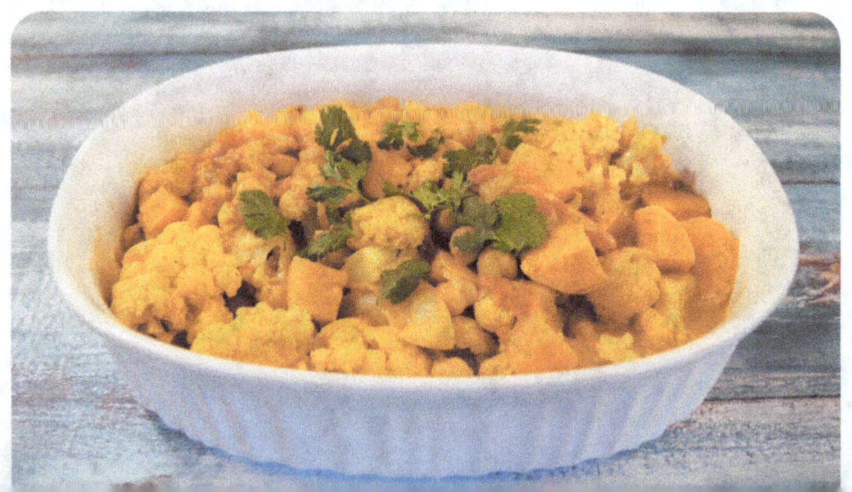

VEGGIE	**Cauliflower Marinara**[V] **Serves 4-6**	**Side**
INGREDIENTS		**SUBSTITUTE**
1	Head cauliflower	
3½ C	Marinara sauce (see Classic Marinara recipe on page 144)	Marinara sauce, one 24 oz jar
1 C	Mozzarella, shredded	Fontina or Parmesan cheese
1 C	Red bell pepper, sliced (optional)	
STEPS		
1	Preheat oven to 375°F. Spray 9" x 13" baking pan with cooking spray.	
2	Cut up cauliflower florets into pieces no thicker than 1½ inches. Arrange cauliflower and red pepper (if using) in pan in a single layer.	
3	Spread Marinara sauce over cauliflower evenly.	
4	Bake in oven for 20 minutes or until you can push a fork into the cauliflower with a little effort (undercooked).	
5	Spread grated cheese over the cauliflower and return to the oven for another 20 minutes.	

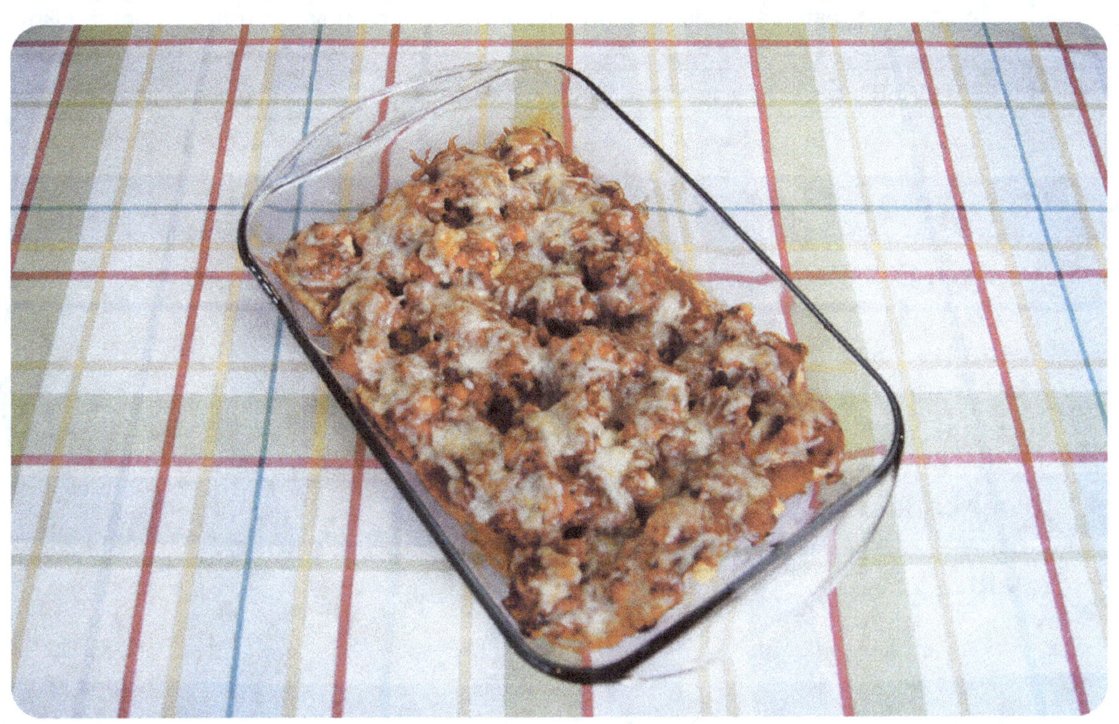

VEGGIE	**Citrus Brussels Sprouts**[V] **Serves 4**	**Side**
INGREDIENTS		**SUBSTITUTE**
1 lb	Brussels sprouts, fresh	Frozen Brussels sprouts
2 Tbsp	Extra Virgin Olive Oil	
2 Tbsp	Butter	
2 Tbsp	Orange juice concentrate	
2 Tbsp	Brown sugar	White sugar or honey
	Salt and pepper to taste	
STEPS		
1	Preheat oven to 400°F. Line a sheet pan with parchment if desired.	
2	Prepare fresh sprouts by cleaning well and cutting in half. If using frozen, leave them whole.	
3	In a bowl, toss the sprouts with the oil to coat them. Put them on the sheet pan in a single layer.	
4	Roast the sprouts for 30-40 minutes, stirring them once after about 20 minutes. Remove from the oven once they are tender.	
5	In a small sauce pan, bring the butter, orange juice concentrate and brown sugar to a boil.	
6	Combine the roasted sprouts and the sauce in a serving bowl, stirring to coat the Brussels sprouts.	

Brussels sprouts interesting facts:

- A cup of Brussels sprouts has 35 calories, 3 g of fiber, and 3 g of protein.
- Contains four times more vitamin C than oranges.
- Stay fresh in the refrigerator vegetable drawer for up to 10 days.
- They contain sulforaphane that has been shown to help lower cancer risks.
- Contain zeaxanthine, an antioxidant, that is good for eye health.

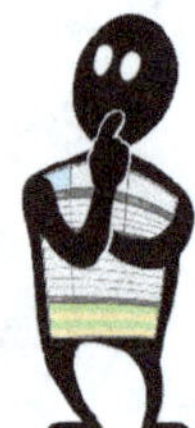

PROTEIN OTHER	**Continental Beans**[V] **Makes ~ 2 cups**	**Side**
INGREDIENTS		**SUBSTITUTE**
2 C	Cooked white beans, drained (15 oz can)	Any cooked or canned beans
2 oz	Bacon, diced (optional)	Pancetta or ham, diced
½	Onion, diced	
3 tsp	Garlic, minced	
1 Tbsp	Herbs de Provence	Rosemary + Thyme
1 Tbsp	Lemon juice	Vinegar
½ Tbsp	Dijon mustard	
2 Tbsp	Olive oil	
STEPS		
1	Cook bacon in a sauté pan until almost crisp, remove from pan for later.	
2	Remove all but 2 Tbsp of bacon grease from pan.	
3	Cook onion in fat from bacon (or add a little oil if you didn't use bacon) until onion is soft.	
4	Add garlic and herbs to the pan and cook another three minutes.	
5	Add beans and bacon to the pan and mix. Heat thoroughly.	
6	Mix lemon juice, mustard and olive oil together in small cup and drizzle over beans prior to serving.	

VEGGIE	**Creamed Vegetables**[V] **Serves 2-4**	**Side**
INGREDIENTS		**SUBSTITUTE**
3 Tbsp	Butter	
½	Onion, finely minced	
1¼ Tbsp	Flour	
1 C	Milk	Heavy cream or Half & Half
1 tsp	Salt	
1 lb	Vegetables, fresh or frozen	
STEPS		
1	Cook vegetables by boiling on the stove top or microwave, per your preference. Drain well.	
2	In a large skillet, melt the butter and cook the onion over medium heat until it is soft and there is no free moisture.	
3	Add the flour to the pan and cook while stirring for two to three minutes to cook the flour.	
4	Add the milk and stir or whisk vigorously to fully incorporate. Continue to heat while stirring until the mixture almost boils and the sauce thickens. Add salt.	
5	Stir the cooked and drained vegetables into the sauce. Add a tablespoon of milk if the sauce is too thick.	
OPTIONS		
A	**Peas:** Make plain or add 2 oz of grated Parmesan cheese and a ¼ tsp of nutmeg to the sauce before combining with peas.	
B	**Potatoes**: Use small red or fingerling potatoes, cut into halves. Multiply the sauce recipe by the number of pounds of potatoes. If desired, add 1 C grated cheese to the sauce.	
C	**Cauliflower**: Cut one head of cauliflower (about 2 pounds) into florets before cooking. Double the amount of sauce and add 1 C grated cheese to the sauce if desired.	
D	**Spinach**: After cooking the spinach, squeeze to remove as much water as possible. Add 2 oz of grated parmesan cheese and a ¼ tsp of nutmeg to the sauce before combining.	
E	**Corn**: Start with fresh or frozen corn, cook and drain well. Add 1 tsp of sugar and ¼ tsp black pepper to the sauce before combining.	
F	**Mixed**: Combine any two veggies (e.g. peas + cauliflower, peas + potatoes, corn + green beans). Multiply the sauce recipe by the number of pounds of veggies.	

VEGGIE	Frizzled Cabbage[V] Makes about 3-5 cups	Side
INGREDIENTS		**SUBSTITUTE**
1-1½ lb	Cabbage, sliced finely	Red or green cabbage, fresh or bag
1-2 Tbsp	Extra Virgin Olive Oil	Bacon fat or butter or any oil
2 - 4	Slices of bacon, chopped (optional)	Finely chopped ham or pancetta
½ C	Onion and/or red pepper, sliced (optional)	
½ - 1 C	Carrot, shredded (optional)	
1 tsp	Salt and pepper, each	
2 Tbsp	Butter, as dressing	2-3 Tbsp Tahini or 4-6 Tbsp sour cream

STEPS	
1	If using bacon, cook in large skillet until crispy. Remove bacon and leave fat in pan.
2	Sauté cabbage and any other veggies in the oil (or bacon fat) over medium high heat, stirring often, until tender and beginning to caramelize. About 15 minutes.
3	Salt and pepper to taste. Toss with butter (or Tahini or sour cream) prior to serving.
4	Top with crumbled bacon, if using.

OPTIONS	
A	**Simply Savory**: Recipe above - plain red or green cabbage with salt, pepper and butter.
B	**Colorful and Complex:** Cabbage, onions, pepper and carrots frizzled to a nice caramelized tenderness. Stir in Tahini prior to serving for a rich and satisfying taste.
C	**Creamy:** Frizzle the cabbage then stir in sour cream prior to serving. Particularly good with a crispy pancetta or bacon garnish.

VEGGIE	**Glazed Carrots**[V] **Serves 4**	**Side**
INGREDIENTS		**SUBSTITUTE**
1 lb	Carrots, any type	
2 Tbsp	Butter	Extra Virgin Olive Oil
2 Tbsp	Brown sugar	Maple syrup, honey
½ tsp	Cinnamon	Ginger
STEPS		
1	Peel and cut carrots so that they are uniform in shape and thickness. Can be sticks or coins or can use bagged baby carrots.	
2	Boil carrots in water until tender – about 6-10 minutes depending on thickness.	
3	Drain carrots well and set aside. The serving bowl works well.	
4	Put remaining ingredients into the pan and heat over medium heat, stirring to combine.	
5	When the glaze is bubbly, return the carrots to the pan. Stir over medium heat for several minutes to glaze the carrots.	
OPTIONS		
A	**Orange Ginger**: Add 1 Tbsp orange juice concentrate to the glaze mixture and replace the cinnamon with 1 tsp ginger paste or ½ tsp dried ginger.	
B	**Maple Bourbon**: Add 1 Tbsp bourbon to the glaze mixture and replace brown sugar with maple syrup.	
C	**Sweet & Spicy**: Replace cinnamon with ½ tsp red pepper flakes and ¼ tsp salt.	

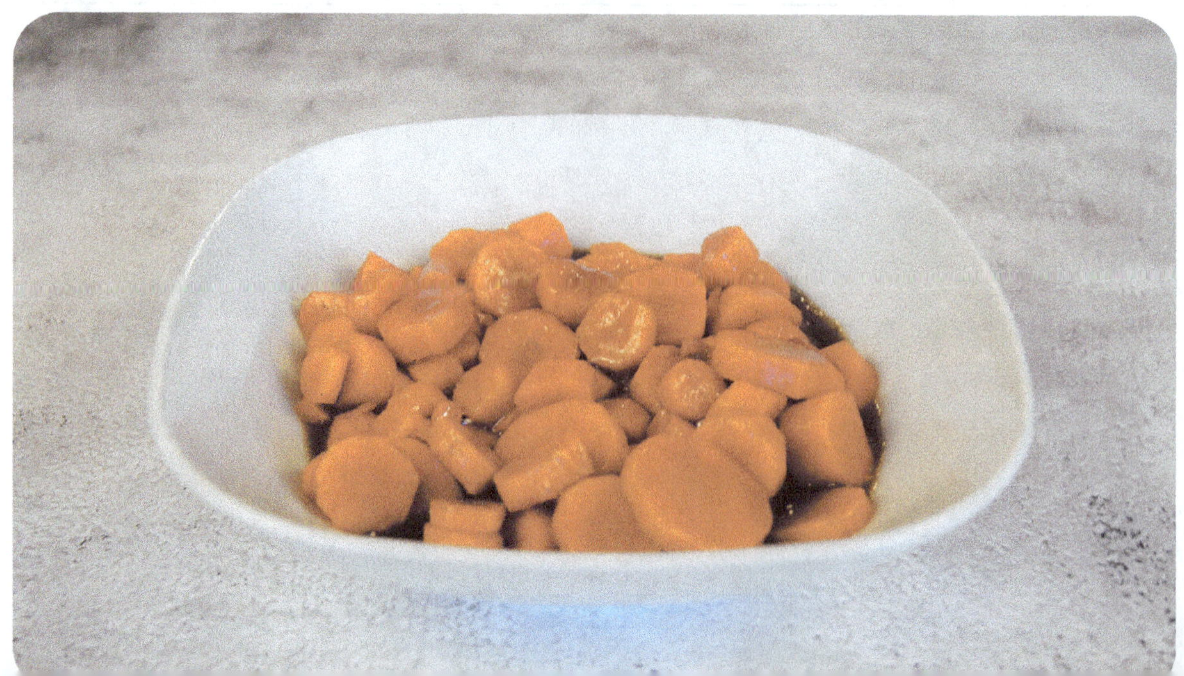

VEGGIE	Green Beans[V] Serves 2-4	Side
INGREDIENTS		**SUBSTITUTE**
1 lb	Green beans, whole	Frozen green beans
2 Tbsp	Extra Virgin Olive Oil	Butter
4	Cloves garlic, minced	2 tsp jarred minced garlic
¼ tsp	Red pepper flakes	
STEPS		
1	Steam or microwave green beans until they are tender-crisp, slightly less than done. Drain.	
2	In a sauté pan, cook the garlic and pepper flakes in the oil or butter for 1-2 minutes.	
3	Add the cooked green beans to the pan and toss over medium heat to thoroughly coat the green beans. Salt to taste and serve.	
OPTIONS		
A	**Almondine**: Garnish with ½ C sliced almonds.	
B	**Mushroom**: Add 8 oz of sautéed mushrooms to the garlic and oil, then toss with the green beans.	
C	**Italian**: Add ½ of a sautéed sliced red pepper and ½ tsp oregano or basil to the garlic and oil, then toss with the green beans.	
D	**Asian**: Sauté 1 tsp ginger paste with the garlic. Add 2 Tbsp soy sauce and 1 Tbsp honey when tossing the green beans.	

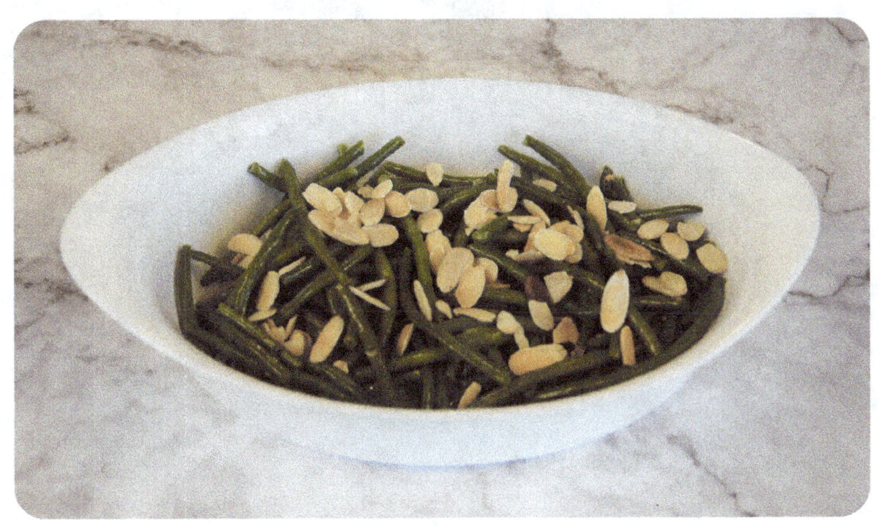

VEGGIE	**Green Bean Succotash**[V] **Serves 4-6**	**Side**
INGREDIENTS		**SUBSTITUTE**
1 lb	Green beans, whole fresh	Frozen
12 oz	Sweet corn, cut from cob	Frozen
2 Tbsp	Butter	Extra Virgin Olive Oil
½	Red bell pepper, thinly sliced (optional)	
1 C	Cherry tomatoes, halved (optional)	
STEPS		
1	Put green beans and corn in a pot together and add 1 cup of water. Bring water to a boil then cook for about eight minutes or until desired doneness. Drain.	
2	If including bell pepper, sauté it in the butter for about four minutes.	
3	Add the cooked green beans, corn, and cherry tomatoes (if using) to the pan and stir together over medium heat for 1-2 minutes to thoroughly mix. Salt to taste and serve.	

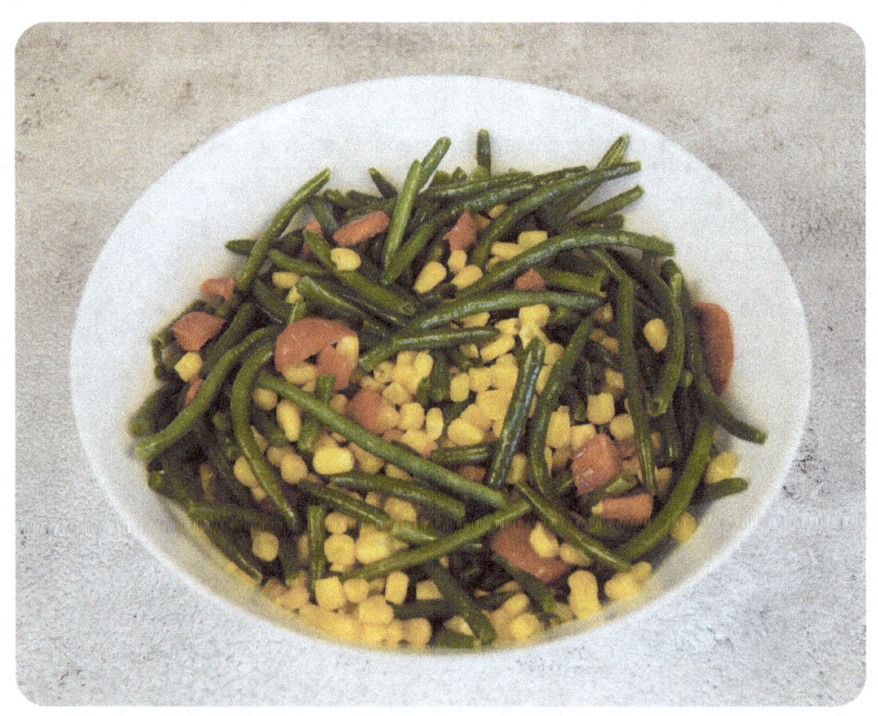

VEGGIE	Green Bean Un-Casserole^V Makes 4 cups	Side
INGREDIENTS		**SUBSTITUTE**
1 lb	Green beans, trimmed	Frozen green beans
1½ Tbsp	Butter	Extra Virgin Olive Oil, olive or other light oil
1 Tbsp	Flour	
1 C	Milk	
½ Tbsp	Dehydrated onion flakes	2 Tbsp diced onion + 2 tsp oil microwaved together for 20 seconds on high (covered)
1 Tbsp	Mushroom or Umami seasoning	1 Tbsp mushroom powder + 1 tsp salt
½ C	Bread crumbs (optional)	
STEPS		
1	Put green beans in a sauce pan with one cup of water and cover. Bring to a boil and then cook for five to seven minutes to desired tenderness. Drain and set aside.	
2	In a sauté pan, melt butter and add flour. Cook over medium heat and allow to bubble while stirring for two to three minutes to make a light roux.	
3	Add milk to pan, stirring continuously. Bring mixture to almost a boil so that the sauce thckens.	
4	Remove from heat and add onion flakes and mushroom seasoning.	
5	Toss green beans with the onion / mushroom sauce.	
6	Top with bread crumbs (optional) then serve.	

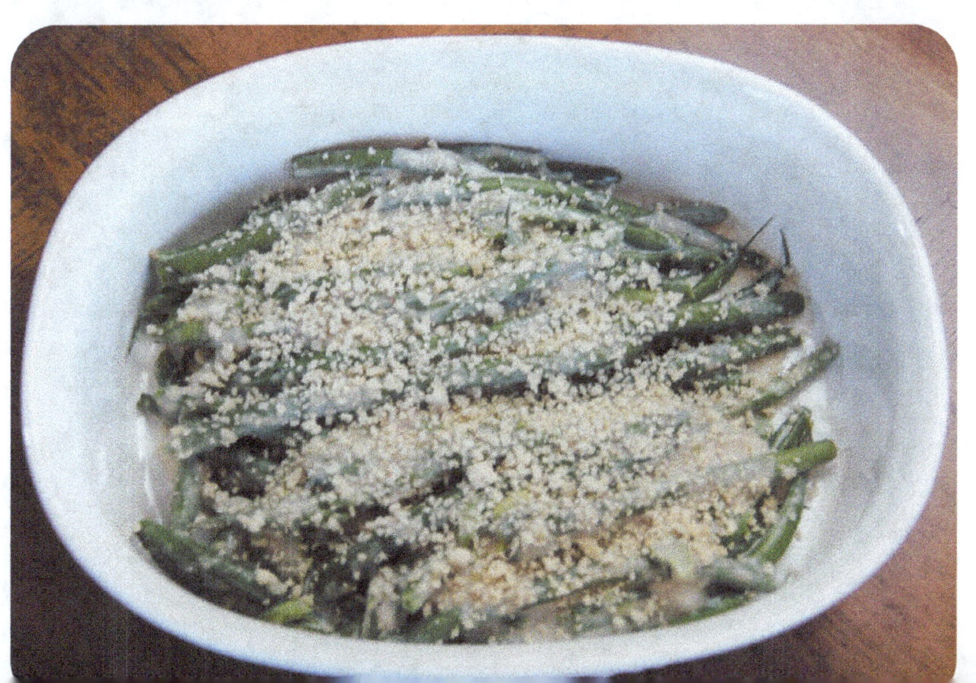

VEGGIE	**Lemon Bacon Brussels Sprouts**^{V} **Serves 4-6**	**Side**
INGREDIENTS		**SUBSTITUTE**
1½ ibs	Brussels sprouts	
3-4 slices	Bacon, diced	
1	Lemon, cut into ¼ inch thick slices	
1 tsp	Salt	
STEPS		
1	Preheat oven to 400°F.	
2	Prepare Brussels sprouts by cleaning and cutting into halves.	
3	In an large oven proof skillet, sauteé bacon until crispy and fat has rendered.	
4	Add sprouts to the pan with the bacon and fat. Allow them to brown over medium high heat for three to four minutes, then stir/turn them to brown on the other side for another three to four minutes.	
5	Add salt and lemon slices, stirring just enough to evenly distribute through the sprouts.	
6	Bake for 10-15 minutes, or to desired tenderness.	

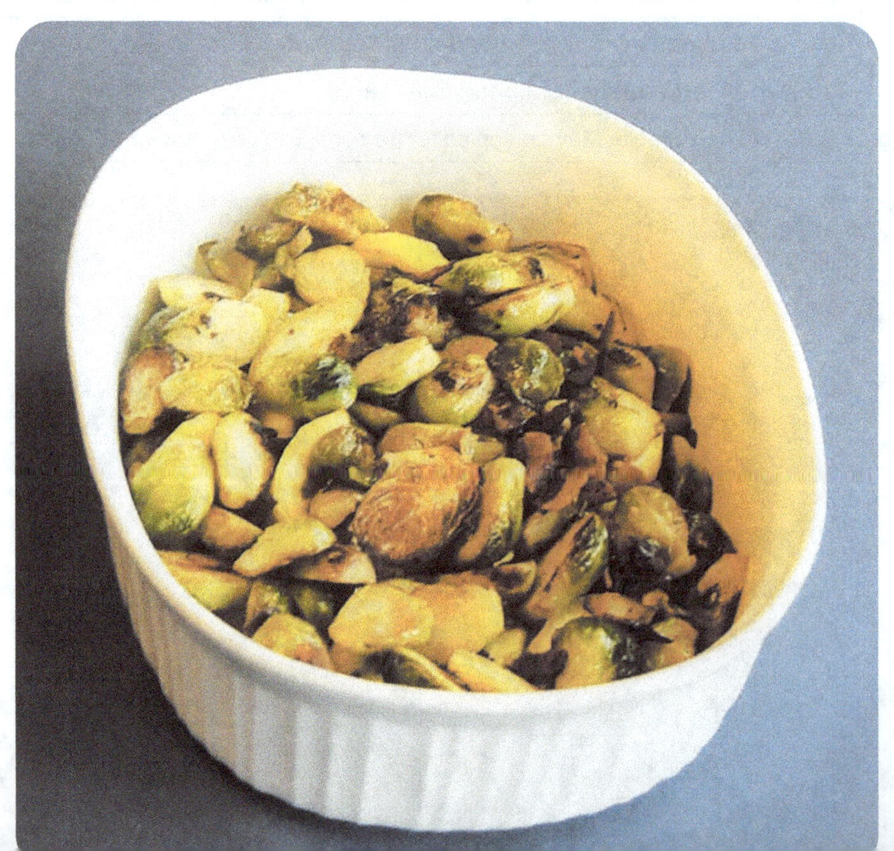

VEGGIE	Lemon Garlic Kale[V] Serves 2-4	Side
INGREDIENTS		**SUBSTITUTE**
1 bunch	Fresh kale (about 9 oz)	
2 Tbsp	Extra Virgin Olive Oil	Any olive or light cooking oil
3 - 4	Garlic cloves, minced	Jarred minced garlic
1 tsp	Stock paste or bouillon powder	
½ C	Water	
1 Tbsp	Lemon juice	
1 Tbsp	Butter	Margarine
1 Tbsp	Grated Paremesan cheese (optional)	
STEPS		
1	Prepare kale by washing well in cold water and then remove stems and slice leaves.	
2	In a large sauce pan, sauté garlic in olive oil for two minutes.	
3	Add water and stock paste to the pan and then stir in kale.	
4	Cover the pan and cook over medium heat for about six minutes until kale leaves are tender.	
5	Stir in the lemon juice and butter, and continue to cook uncovered until liquid is mostly gone.	
6	Serve plain or with a garnish of grated parmesan cheese.	

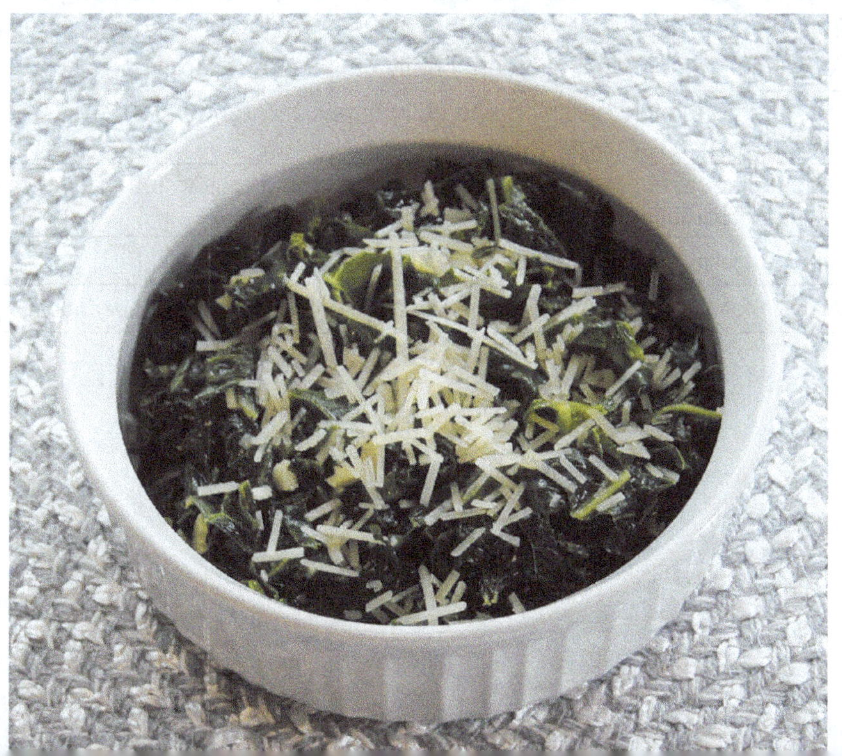

VEGGIE	Mediterranean Spaghetti Squash^V Serves 4-6	Side
INGREDIENTS		**SUBSTITUTE**
1	Spaghetti squash (about 1½ lbs)	Summer squash, julienne cut
2 Tbsp	Extra Virgin Olive Oil	Olive oil, butter, or any light cooking oil
1	Onion, sliced (red)	Any onion
1	Red bell pepper, sliced	
1	Medium tomato, diced	Cherry tomatoes, halved
1 Tbsp	Oregano	
1 tsp	Salt	
2-4 oz	Feta, crumbled	
STEPS		
1	Remove the stem and cut the squash in half long wise. Scrape out and dispose of the seeds and associated strings.	
2	Place one half squash face down on a flat microwave safe plate or pan. Depending on the size of your microwave and available pans, you may need to cook the halves sequentially.	
3	For one half squash, microwave on high for seven minutes. Test for doneness by pressing on the outside (with an oven glove): if you can easily form a dent, the squash is done.	
4	If not done yet, continue to cook on high in two minute increments until the flesh is tender and readily gives when pressed.	
5	Carefully scrape the squash fibers out of the shell using a fork, separating and fluffing them as you go. The cooked squash can be held at this point for later use.	
6	If you are using summer squash, steam briefly until tender crisp.	
7	In a large sauté pan, cook the onion and bell pepper until tender. Add the tomatoes and cook for another one to two minutes.	
8	Add the cooked squash, oregano and salt to the pan and toss together over medium heat for a two minutes to combine and warm.	
9	Serve with the crumbled feta on top.	

Photo on page 169

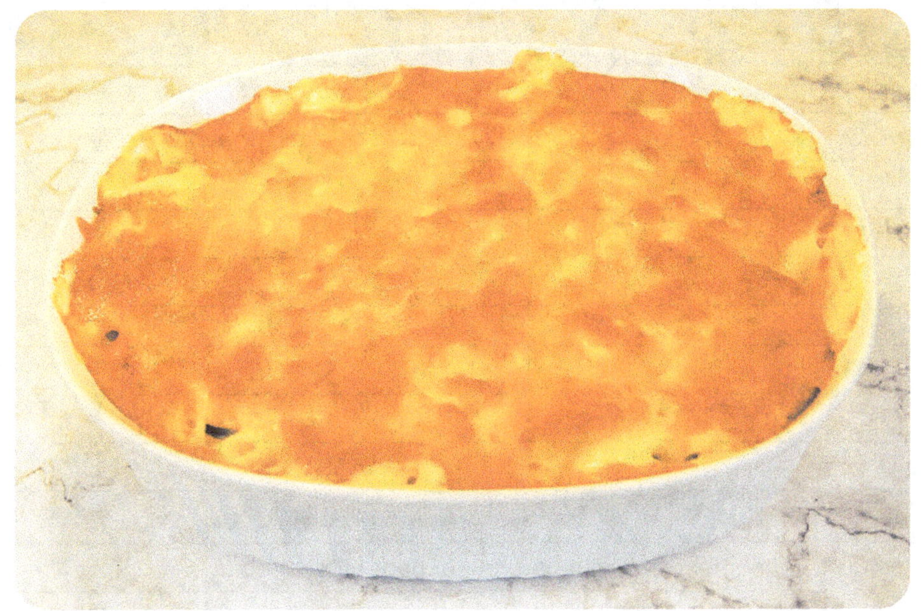

$100 Mac & Cheese

Recipe on page 152

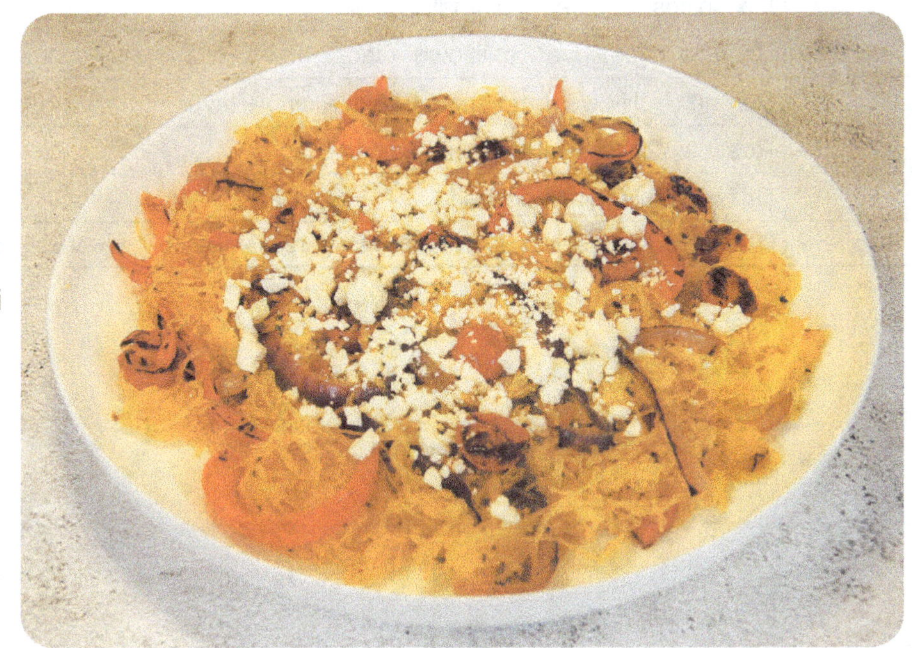

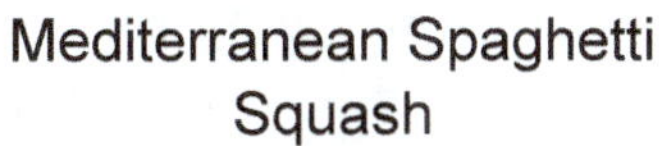

Mediterranean Spaghetti Squash

Recipe on page 168

VEGGIE	**Moroccan Cauliflower[V]** **Serves 2-4**	**Side**
INGREDIENTS		**SUBSTITUTE**
1	Head cauliflower	
3 Tbsp	Extra Virgin Olive Oil	Olive oil, coconut oil, or avocado oil
½ tsp	Turmeric	
1 tsp	Cumin	
1 tsp	Paprika	
1 tsp	Salt	
1 tsp	Cinnamon	
½ tsp	Clove	
2 Tbsp	Tahini (optional)	
STEPS		
1	Preheat oven to 400°F. Line sheet pan with parchment paper if desired.	
2	Cut cauliflower into florets approximately one to two inches in size.	
3	In a bowel, toss the cauliflower pieces with oil to coat.	
4	Mix spices together in a small bowel.	
5	Sprinkle spices over cauliflower pieces and turn to evenly distribute.	
6	Spread cauliflower onto sheet pan in a single layer.	
7	Roast for 20-30 minutes, until tender-crisp.	
8	Drizzle with Tahini if desired.	

FRUIT	Pineapple Casserole[V] Serves 6-8	Side
INGREDIENTS		**SUBSTITUTE**
1	20 oz can crushed pineapple in juice	Pineapple in syrup - omit sugar
⅔ C	Brown sugar	White sugar or any dry sugar substitute
½ tsp	Salt	
4 Tbsp	Flour	4 Tbsp cornstarch
3	Eggs, large or larger	
1½ C	Bread crumbs, plain dry	2 C soft bread cubes
8 Tbsp	Melted butter	
STEPS		
1	Preheat oven to 350°F. Prepare a 1½ Qt baking dish by coating it with oil or butter.	
2	Mix the pinapple and juice with salt, sugar and flour.	
3	Add the eggs and mix well. Stir in the bread crumbs.	
4	Stir in 6 Tbsp of melted butter, reserving 2 Tbsp for the top.	
5	Pour into baking dish and drizzle the remaing 2 Tbsp of butter over the top.	
6	Bake for 40-50 minutes until hot (at least 160° F) and the top is golden.	
7	Serve as a side; compliments ham, roasted meat, or fowl very nicely.	
OPTIONS		
A	**Dessert:** Add ½ C dried fruit or nuts then serve with a sweet sauce such as caramel or the orange honey ginger sauce on pages 142 and 143.	

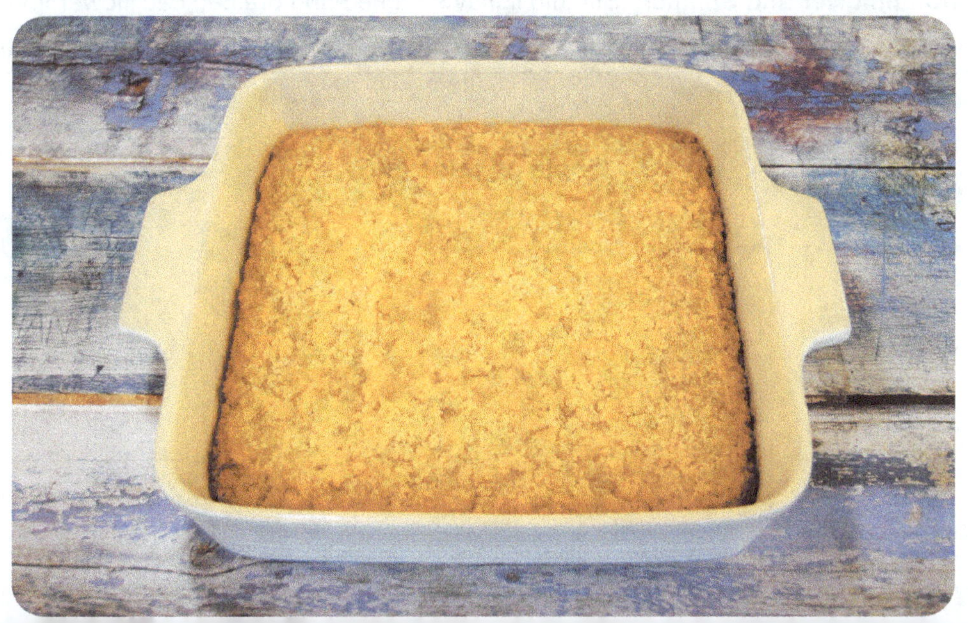

VEGGIE	**Quick Creamed Spinach^{V}** **Serves 2-4**	**Side**
INGREDIENTS		**SUBSTITUTE**
1 lb	Frozen chopped spinach	Fresh spinach
4 oz	Cream cheese	Neufchatel or goat cheese
½ tsp	Dehydrated onion	¼ tsp onion powder
⅛ tsp	Nutmeg (optional)	
½ tsp	Salt (optional)	
1 Tbsp	Grated Parmesan cheese (optional)	
STEPS		
1	Cook frozen spinach according to package directions. If using fresh spinach, saute in olive oil until wilted.	
2	Press excess water out of spinach by pressing it against the side of the pan with a fork. Drain water.	
3	Add onion and cream cheese to cooked spinach. Allow to melt in warm pan.	
4	Stir to incorporate the melting cream cheese. Use low heat if necessary.	
5	Add nutmeg and salt if desired. Garnish with grated Parmasean.	
OPTIONS		
A	**Side Dish**: Creamed spinach is always an elegant side dish served alone.	
B	**Pasta Florentine**: Toss with 8 oz cooked pasta and ½ C pasta water. Serve with a generous garnish of Parmesan cheese.	
C	**Chicken Florentine**: Dress up pan-sautéed chicken breast with a few tablespoons of creamed spinach on top.	
D	**Cauliflower and Spinach**: Stir into lightly steamed and drained cauliflower florets.	

Photo on page 176

VEGGIE	**Quick Spaghetti Squash**[V] **Serves 4-6**	**Side**
INGREDIENTS		**SUBSTITUTE**
1	Spaghetti squash (about 1½ lbs)	
2 Tbsp	Butter	Extra Virgin Olive Oil
2 Tbsp	Orange juice concentrate	1 Tbsp lemon or lime juice
2 Tbsp	Sugar, white	Honey, brown sugar
1 tsp	Salt	
1 Tbsp	Parsley (optional)	

STEPS	
1	Remove the stem and cut the squash in half long wise. Scrape out and dispose of the seeds and associated strings.
2	Place one half squash face down on a flat microwave safe plate or pan. Depending on the size of your microwave and available pans, you may need to cook the halves sequentially.
3	For one half squash, microwave on high for seven minutes. Test for doneness by pressing on the outside (with an oven glove): if you can easily form a dent, the squash is done.
4	If not done yet, continue to cook on high in two minute increments until the flesh is tender and readily gives when pressed.
5	Carefully scrape the squash fibers out of the shell using a fork, separating and fluffing them as you go. The cooked squash can be held at this point for later use.
6	In a large sauté pan, stir the butter, orange juice concentrate, sugar and salt together over medium heat.
7	Add the cooked squash to the pan and toss to warm and coat it. Serve with a garnish of parsley if desired.

GRAIN	Rice Pilaf^V Serves 2-4	Side
INGREDIENTS		**SUBSTITUTE**
4 C	Cooked rice	
2 Tbsp	Extra Virgin Olive Oil	Butter, any light oil
1	Onion, diced	
2	Cloves garlic	1 tsp minced jarred garlic
8-16 oz	Mushrooms, sliced	Peas, spinach, broccoli
1 Tbsp	Basil	Thyme, oregano
1 tsp	Salt	
1 C	Grated cheese (optional)	
STEPS		
1	In a large pot, sauté the onion in the oil until soft. Add the garlic and cook an additional minute.	
2	Add the mushrooms and cook until the moisture is nearly gone. Stir in the salt and spices.	
3	Add the cooked rice to the pot and stir to incorporate. If the rice is cold, you can add 2 Tbsp of water to the pot, cover over low heat for three to five minutes to warm it.	
4	When the rice is hot, you can serve it directly or topped with grated cheese.	
5	If desired, the pilaf can be put in a casserole dish with cheese on top and then baked for 10-15 minutes at 350°F, until the cheese is melted and golden.	
OPTIONS		
A	**Mushroom Pilaf**: Recipe as above. Swiss cheese goes well with the mushrooms.	
B	**Risi Bisi**: Replace the mushrooms with two cups cooked peas. Top with Parmesan cheese.	
C	**Tuscan Pilaf**: Replace the mushrooms with 16 oz spinach, cooked and squeezed dry. Add ½ C diced sun dried tomatoes (in oil) and ½ C of pine nuts. Top with Parmesan cheese.	
D	**Broccoli Cheddar**: Replace the mushrooms with two cups of cooked broccoli florets. Stir in one cup of sharp cheddar cheese and then top with another cup of cheese.	

Photo on page 176

VEGGIE	**Roasted Vegetables^V** **Serves 4-8**	**Side**
INGREDIENTS		**SUBSTITUTE**
2 lb	Mixed vegetables: Carrots, potatoes, onions, cauliflower, broccoli, peppers, sweet potatoes	Butternut squash, Brussels sprouts, summer squash, beets
2 Tbsp	Extra Virgin Olive Oil	Melted butter
1 tsp	Salt	
½ tsp	Cracked black pepper	
STEPS		
1	Preheat oven to 400°F.	
2	Prepare the vegetables by cutting them into uniform size pieces, no thicker than one inch.	
3	Place the more dense veggies (carrots, cauliflower, potatoes, etc.) in a large bowl and toss with olive oil and spices.	
4	Spread these veggies on a large sheet pan and put in the oven for 25 minutes.	
5	Place the less dense veggies (broccoli, onions, peppers, etc.) in a large bowl and toss with the remaining olive oil and spices.	
6	Remove the sheet pan from the oven and stir. Add the less dense veggies and roast for an additional 20-30 minutes, or until desired level of doneness.	
7	If you increase the recipe, use additional sheet pans so that the veggies can roast in a single layer.	
OPTIONS		
A	**Savory**: Mix 1 tsp minced garlic and 2 tsp Herbs de Provence or rosemary into the olive oil before tossing with the veggies.	
B	**Sweet**: Mix 2 Tbsp brown sugar and 1 tsp cinnamon into the oil before tossing with carrots, sweet potatoes or butternut squash.	
C	**Spicy**: Mix 1 tsp minced garlic and ½ tsp each cumin, coriander, paprika and red pepper flakes into the oil before tossing with the veggies.	
D	**Balsamic Glazed**: Mix 1 tsp minced garlic, 1 tsp thyme and ¼ C Balsamic vinegar with the oil before tossing with the veggies.	

Photo on page 176

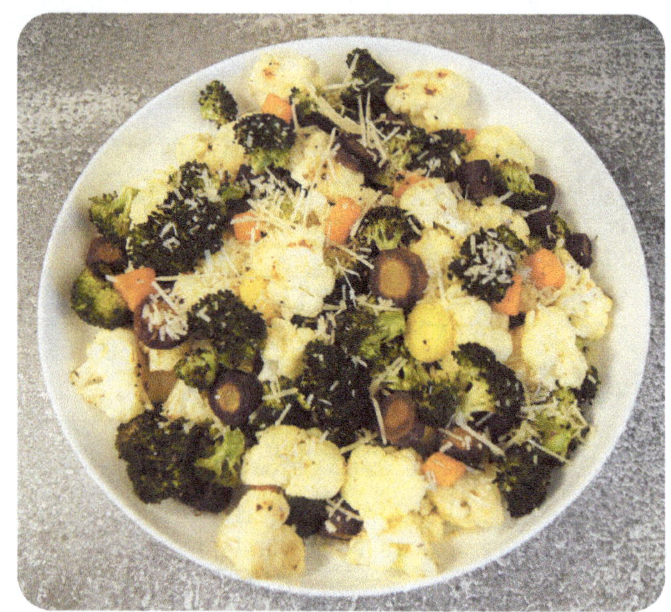

Roasted Vegetables

Recipe on page 175

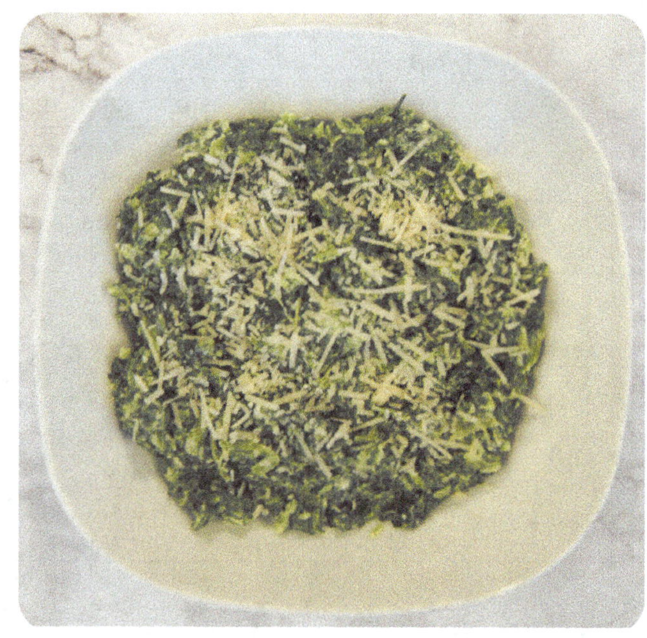

Quick Creamed Spinach

Recipe on page 172

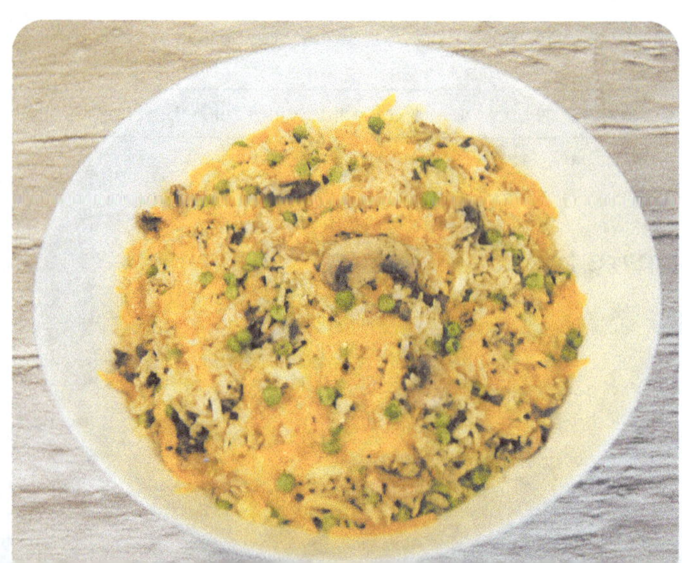

Rice Pilaf w/ Mushrooms and Peas

Recipe on page 174

VEGGIE	**Sautéed Baby Bok Choy[V]** **Serves 2-4**	**Side**
INGREDIENTS		**SUBSTITUTE**
4-6	Heads baby bok choy, halved longways	
2 Tbsp	Canola oil	Any light oil
2	Cloves garlic	1 tsp minced jarred garlic
2	Green onions, sliced	
2 Tbsp	Soy sauce	
1 tsp	Sesame oil	
1 tsp	Honey	
2 Tbsp	Water	
STEPS		
1	In a large fry pan with a lid, heat the oil and garlic and cook for one minute.	
2	Place the bok choy halves, face down in the pan in the hot oil. Cook over medium high heat for two minutes with out stirring so that the face starts to caramelize.	
3	Mix the remaining ingredients and add to pan. Shake the pan to coat the bok choy.	
4	Reduce heat to simmer and cover the pan. Allow to coot for an additional three to five minutes until tender.	

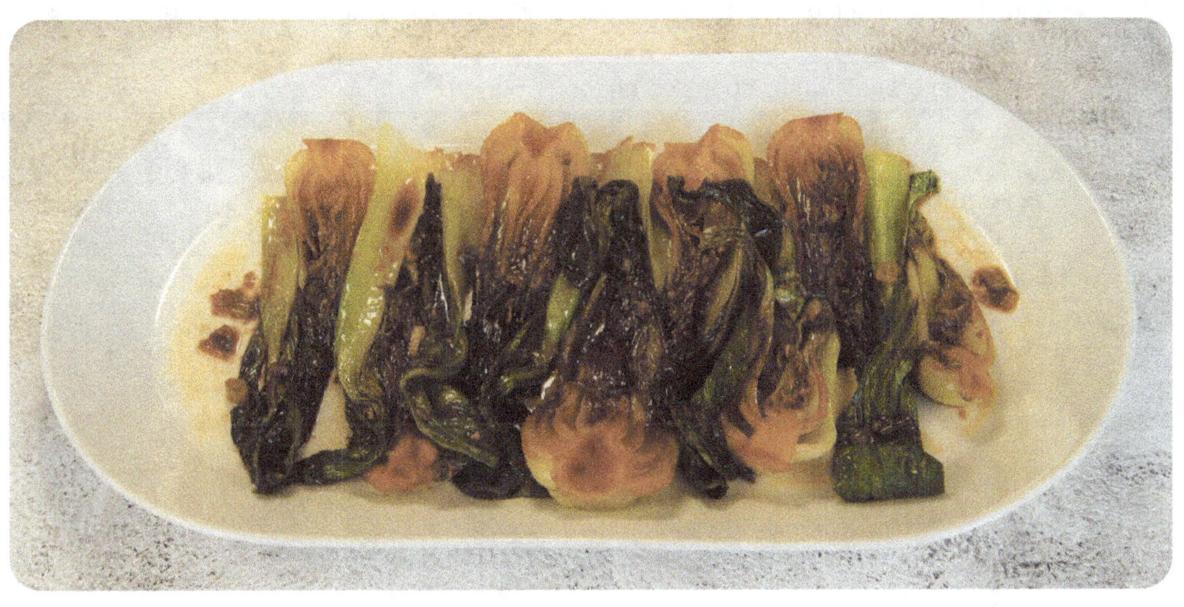

PROTEIN OTHER	Savory White Beans[V] Makes about 2 cups	Side
INGREDIENTS		**SUBSTITUTE**
2	15 oz cans Great Northern Beans, drained	Any canned beans or 4 C of any cooked beans
1	Onion, chopped	
1 tsp	Minced garlic	
3	Carrots, diced	
1 Tbsp	Tomato paste	Ketchup (omit sugar)
1 tsp	Chicken broth base or boullion powder	Vegetable broth base
1 tsp	Herbs de Provence	Thyme + Sage
1 tsp	Salt and black pepper, each	
1 tsp	Sugar	Any sweetener
¼ C	Water	Add more if a thinner consistency is desired
¼ C	Bread crumbs (optional)	Cracker, corn flake, or potato chip crumbs
STEPS		
1	Sauté onion in a sauce pan with a little oil until soft	
2	Add garlic and cook for another few minutes.	
3	Add carrots and water to pan and cook for 8-10 minutes.	
4	Add all remaining ingredients except bread crumbs and simmer for 10 minutes. Add ¼ C water if beans become too dry.	
5	Serve with bread crumbs sprinkled on top.	
OPTIONS		
A	**Casserole**: Make recipe through step 3. Layer beans with 1 lb cooked pork or sausage in a 9" x 9" pan or 1-2 quart casserole dish. Top with crumbs and bake for 30 minutes.	
B	**Soup**: Make recipe through step 3. Add 2 C chicken broth and simmer for 30-60 minutes.	

Photo on page 187

VEGGIE	**Simple Greens[V]** **Serves 2-4**	**Side**
INGREDIENTS		**SUBSTITUTE**
2 lb	Fresh collard greens	Kale, Swiss chard, turnip greens
2 Tbsp	Extra Virgin Olive Oil	Butter, bacon fat, any oil
1	Onion, medium, minced	
2	Cloves garlic	1 tsp minced jarred garlic
2 C	Vegetable or chicken stock	2 C water + 2 tsp stock paste
1 Tbsp	Apple cider vinegar	Any vinegar or lemon juice
1 Tbsp	Sugar, white	Honey, maple syrup
¼ tsp	Red pepper flakes	
STEPS		
1	Prepare greens by thoroughly washing them in cold water. Remove the central stem of each leaf and then slice the leaves into about one inch strips.	
2	In the bottom of a large pan with a lid, sauté the onion in the oil until soft then add the garlic and cook for an additional minute.	
3	Add remaining ingredients and bring to a boil, stirring occasionally.	
4	Reduce heat and simmer covered for 20-45 minutes or until greens are tender. Young, tender greens will cook faster than older, tougher ones.	

Besides being delicious, dark leafy greens like collard greens, kale, Swiss chard, and turnip greens are rich in iron, calcium, magnesium, potassium, and vitamins C, E, and K. They are also an excellent source of fiber and antioxidants.

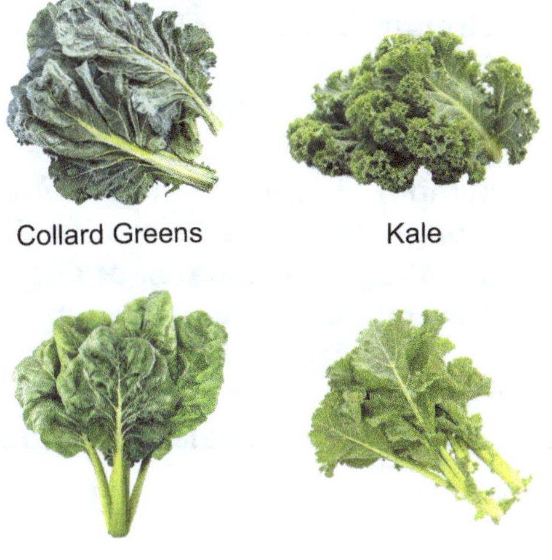

Collard Greens Kale

Swiss Chard Turnip Greens

VEGGIE	Spinach – Flash Sautéed[V] Serves 2-4	Side
INGREDIENTS		**SUBSTITUTE**
6 oz	Fresh spinach leaves	
3 Tbsp	Extra Virgin Olive Oil	Butter
4	Cloves garlic, minced	2 tsp jarred minced garlic
2 Tbsp	Grated Parmesan cheese	
STEPS		
1	Sort and rinse fresh spinach leaves. Dry to remove most of the residual water.	
2	In a large sauté pan, heat the oil and cook the garlic for two to three minutes over medium heat.	
3	Increase heat to medium high and start adding handfuls of spinach leaves. As they wilt, push to the side and add more until all of the spinach is in the pan.	
4	Stir the spinach gently, lifting from below so that it does not become compacted. Cook for about two minutes or until the spinach is uniformly cooked. Salt to taste.	
5	Serve with the parmesan sprinkled on top.	

Spinach and Popeye:

Everyone knows that spinach was Popeye's go to food for strength whenever he got in trouble. Ever wonder why?

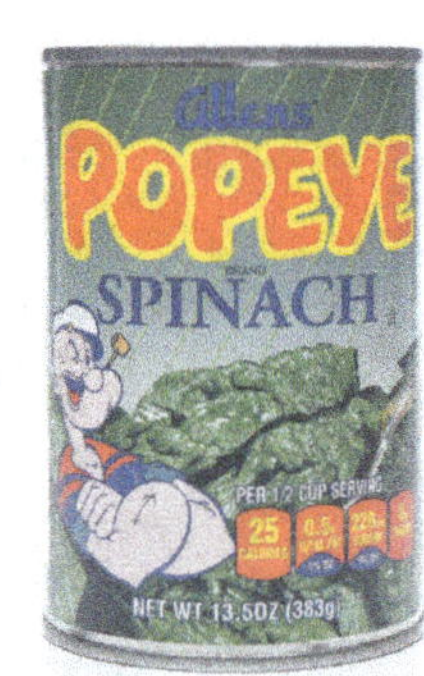

The creator of Popeye read that spinach had a huge amount of iron, 35mg per 100g, so he ran with that and made spinach the symbol of strength in the series. It turns out that there was a typo in the article he read and the actual amount of iron is 3.5mg per 100gm of spinach, or about 20% of the daily recommended amount per serving. Ooops!

During the first four years that the Popeye series ran in the 1930's, spinach sales in the US increased more than 30%.

VEGGIE	**Sweet Potato Casserole^{V}** **Make 8-10 servings**	**Side**
INGREDIENTS		**SUBSTITUTE**
3 lb	Sweet potatoes	
2	Eggs, large or XL	
2 tsp	Vanilla extract	
1 tsp	Cinnamon	
½ tsp	Salt	
1½ C	Brown sugar	White sugar
¼ C	Flour (30 g)	
4 Tbsp	Butter, melted	
¾ C	Chopped pecans or walnuts (optional)	
STEPS		
1	Bake sweet potatoes on a parchment paper lined baking sheet until soft, about one hour at 350°F. Allow sweet potatoes to cool. This step can be done ahead of time.	
2	Preheat oven to 350°F. Generously grease a 9 x 9 inch baking pan or 2½ quart casserole dish.	
3	Scoop out cooked sweet potato meat into a large bowl.	
4	Mix eggs, vanilla extract, salt, cinnamon and ¾ C brown sugar into the sweet potatoes then turn into the prepared pan.	
5	In a small bowl, mix the flour, remaining ¾ C brown sugar, butter and chopped nuts. Spread topping over the sweet potato mixture.	
6	Bake for 35-45 minutes until bubbly and crisp on top. Allow to rest for at least 15 minutes prior to serving.	

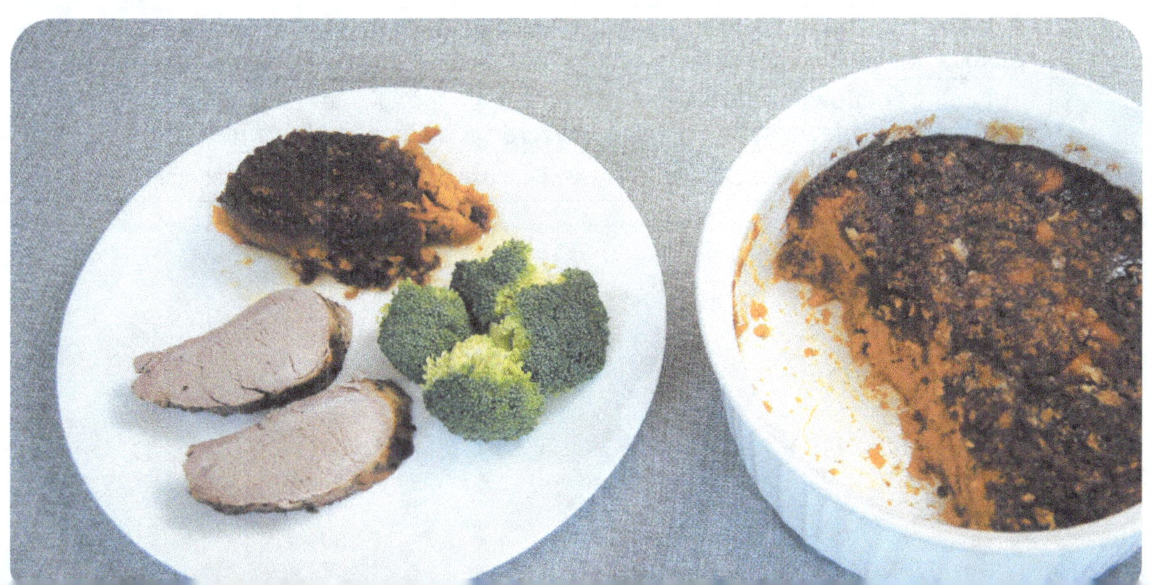

VEGGIE	Vegetables au Gratin[V] Serves 4-6	Side
INGREDIENTS		**SUBSTITUTE**
2½ ib	Potatoes or other vegetable	Carrots, sweet potato, fennel, broccoli, or cauliflower
1	Onion, sliced thin and separated	
1 C	Cheese sauce (see recipe on page 293)	
¼ C	Heavy cream	Half & Half or milk
½ C	Grated cheese (optional)	
	Salt and pepperto taste	
STEPS		
1	Preheat oven to 350°F. Grease a 2 quart baking dish or 9 x 13 pan.	
2	Prepare potatoes or other vegetables by peeling and cutting into thin slices. For root vegetables, slices should be ¼ inch or less.	
3	Prepare cheese sauce as shown on page 293. Cheddar, Swiss, gruyere and parmesan cheeses are all good choices. Salt and pepper to taste.	
4	Stir in an extra ¼ C of cream into the cheese sauce to thin it slightly.	
5	Arrange one layer of vegetables in the pan using ¼ of the vegetables, forming a uniform pattern. Spread ¼ of the onion pieces and top with ¼ of the cheese sauce.	
6	Repeat making layers until the veggies, onion and cheese sauce are used up.	
7	Cover with foil and bake for 30 minutes. Uncover and bake for an additional 20-30 minutes or until the vegetables are tender.	
8	If desired, add a layer of grated cheese on top for the last 10 minutes in the oven.	
OPTIONS		
A	**Potatoes au Gratin**: For best results use Russet potatoes and slice very thin.	
B	**Root Medley**: Use a mix of root vegetables of similar density. Carrots, sweet and white potatoes, fennel bulb are ideas. Use Gruyere, Asiago, Swiss or Parmesan cheese.	
C	**Broccoli Cauliflower au Gratin**: Use one or both for a lighter side dish. Cut into larger slices and make fewer layers. Reduce covered cook time to 15 minutes.	

PROTEIN OTHER	**Bean Soup Express**[V] **Makes about 6 cups**	**Soup**
INGREDIENTS		**SUBSTITUTE**
4 C	Navy beans (two 15 oz cans) drained	Great northern or cannellini beans
1-2	Onions, chopped	
1-2 tsp	Minced garlic	
5	Carrots, diced	
3 Tbsp	Tomato paste	Ketchup
1 Tbsp	Diced parsley	
1 tsp	Thyme	
½ -1 C	Diced ham or pork sausage (optional)	Diced pancetta or cooked bacon: up to ¼ C
1	Potato, diced (optional)	
4 C	Chicken stock	Vegetable stock
	Salt and black pepper to taste	
STEPS		
1	Sauté onion, garlic and carrots in a large sauce pan with a little oil until onion is soft	
2	Add all other ingredients, bring to a boil then simmer for at least 20 minutes. Flavors will develop further if cooked longer.	
3	Meat is optional, but it will add a rich and salty flavor. The optional potato will thicken the soup.	

VEGGIE	**Cream of Mushroom Soup^{V}** **Serves 4-6**	**Soup**
INGREDIENTS		**SUBSTITUTE**
4 Tbsp	Extra Virgin Olive Oil	Butter
2 lb	Mushrooms, sliced or chopped (white or cremini)	Wild mushroom blend
½	Onion, medium, finely diced	Shallots
4	Cloves garlic, minced	2 tsp jarred minced garlic
4 C	Chicken stock (1 qt box)	Vegetable stock
1 tsp	Salt	
½ tsp	Thyme	
½ C	Heavy cream	½ C milk + 2 tsp flour, mixed to a smooth slurry
STEPS		
1	In a large heavy bottomed stock pot, sauté mushrooms and onion until most of the moisture has evaporated.	
2	Stir in the garlic and cook for another two minutes.	
3	Add stock, salt and thyme and simmer for 20-30 minutes.	
4	Remove from heat and blend the soup using a heat resistant immersion blender. A counter top blender could be used, exercising great care in handling the hot liquid.	
5	Return to low heat and stir in the heavy cream. If you are using the milk/flour slurry, continue stirring over low heat until the soup thickens slightly.	
6	Serve plain or garnished with chives or croutons.	

VEGGIE	**French Onion Soup**[V] **Serves 4**	**Soup**
INGREDIENTS		**SUBSTITUTE**
4 Tbsp	Butter	Extra Virgin Olive Oil
3	Onions, medium, sliced thin	Sweet or yellow onions preferred
½ tsp	Salt and pepper, each	
2 tsp	Sugar	
1 C	White wine, dry	Dry red wine
4 C	Beef stock (one 32 oz box)	Vegetable or mushroom stock
1 tsp	Herbs de Provence	Thyme
½	Baguette, sliced into 8 discs	Any bread, sliced
4 oz	Aged Swiss cheese, grated	Gruyere or Emmentaler or Parmesan cheese

STEPS	
1	In a large, heavy bottomed pot, sauté onions in the butter over medium heat until soft.
2	Add salt, pepper and sugar to the onions and reduce heat to medium low. Continue to cook until onions are caramelized, stirring occasionally – about a half hour.
3	Add wine to onions and cook over medium heat to reduce liquid by half.
4	Add stock and herbs. Simmer for at least 20 minutes.
5	Place bread slices on a cookie sheet and top with grated cheese.
6	Broil bread and cheese until melty and crisp.
7	Serve soup in four bowls, each with two to three cheese toasts floating on top.

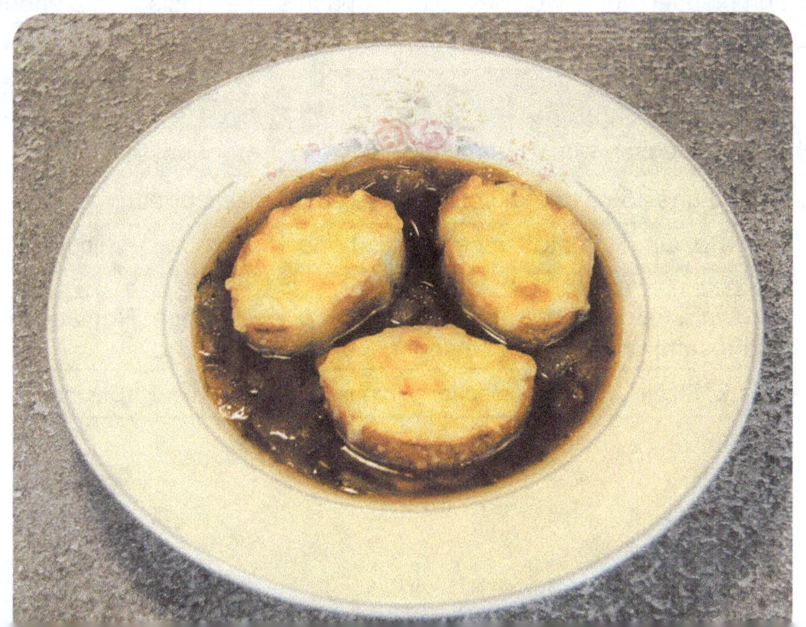

PROTEIN OTHER	**Lentil Soup[V]** **Makes about 6 cups**	**SOUP**
INGREDIENTS		**SUBSTITUTE**
1⅓ C	Lentils, brown, red or green	
1 Tbsp	Extra Virgin Olive Oil	Any olive or light cooking oil
1	Onion, small, diced	
1 tsp	Garlic, minced	
2 tsp	Ginger paste	Grated fresh ginger root
32 oz	Chicken broth (one 32 oz box)	Vegetable broth, water + 4 tsp bullion
1 C	Water	
2 C	Chopped spinach or kale (optional)	Fresh or frozen
8 oz	Tomato sauce	2 Tbsp tomato paste + 7 oz water
2 tsp	Cumin	
3	Carrots, cut into coins (optional)	
1 tsp	Salt	
STEPS		
1	Rinse and sort lentils per package directions.	
2	Sauté onion in olive oil over medium heat until soft. Add garlic and ginger paste and cook for another minute or two.	
3	Add remaining ingredients and bring to a boil.	
4	Reduce heat to simmer and cover. Cook over low heat until lentils are tender, about 45 minutes. If soup seems too thick, add one cup of water.	
5	If you prefer a creamier texture, smash some the of the lentils. A few bursts with an immersion blender works well or you can smash some lentils with a spoon.	
6	Serve plain or with a dollop of sour cream or yogurt and chopped cilantro.	
OPTIONS		
A	**Curry**: Replace cumin with 1 Tbsp curry powder or curry paste.	
B	**Creamy**: Add one 15 oz can of coconut milk to the basic or curry recipe.	
C	**Spicy Tomato**: Omit tomato sauce and add one 15.5 oz can of diced tomatoes and 1 tsp red pepper flakes. Can be added to basic, curry or creamy recipes.	
D	**Meaty**: Brown a few ounces of bacon, ham, or pork sausage. Replace ginger and cumin with thyme and rosemary. Serve with a sprinkle of Parmesan cheese.	

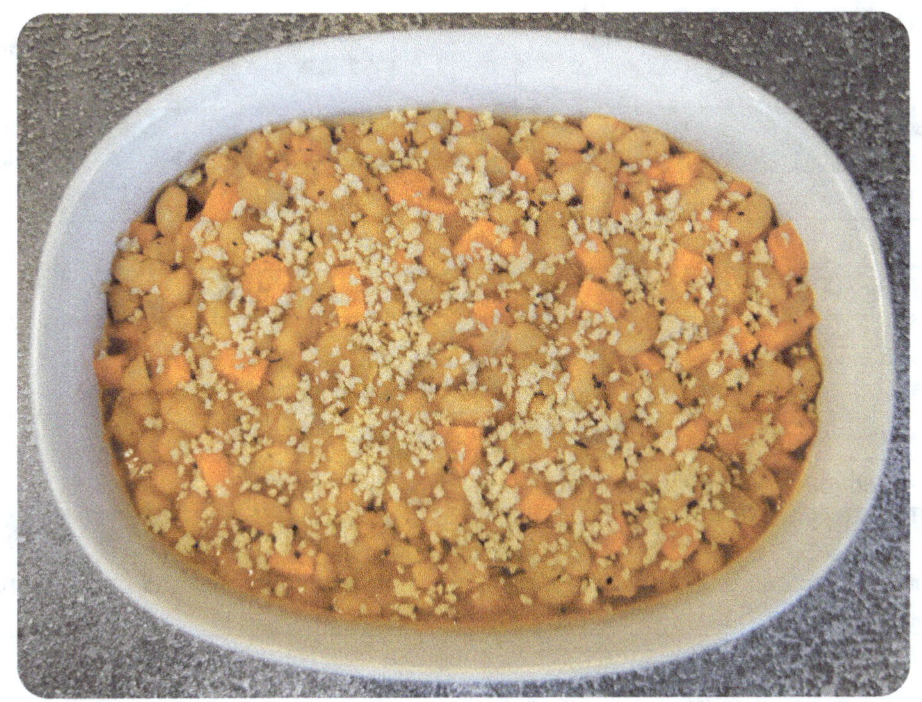

Savory White Beans

Recipe on page 178

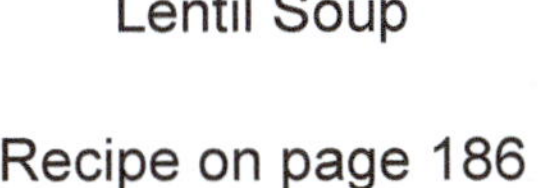

Lentil Soup

Recipe on page 186

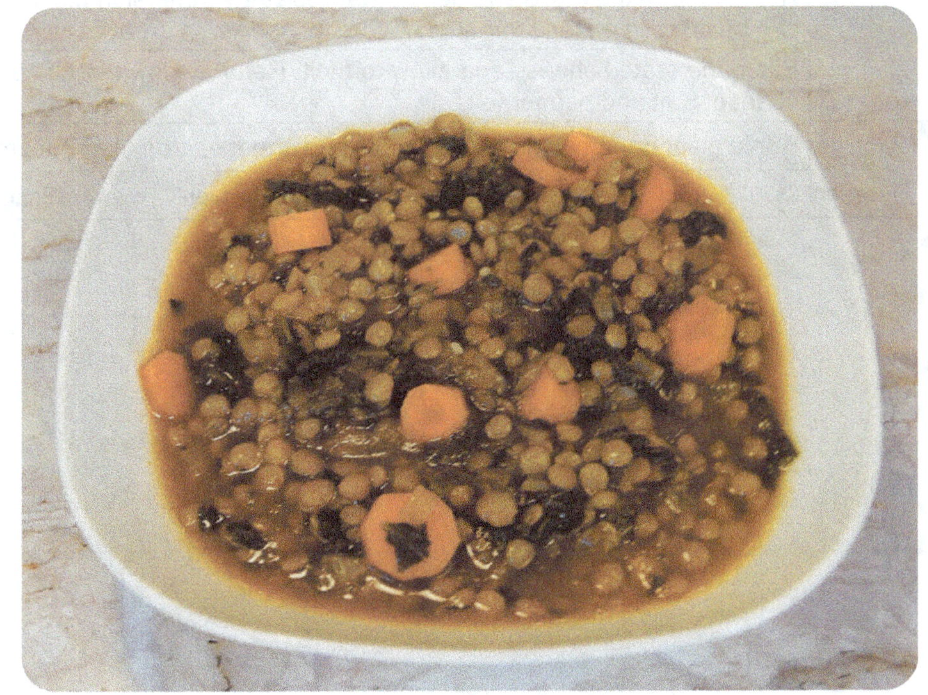

VEGGIE	**Potato Broccoli Soup[V]** **Serves 4-6**	**Soup**
INGREDIENTS		**SUBSTITUTE**
2 Tbsp	Butter	Light cooking oil
1	Onion, finely diced	
4	Cloves garlic, minced	2 tsp minced jarred garlic
1 lb	Potatoes, diced	
4-5 C	Broccoli florets (about 2 stalks)	Frozen broccoli florets
32 oz	Chicken or vegetable broth	
2 C	Grated cheese, cheddar or Co-Jack	
STEPS		
1	In a stock pot, melt the butter and sauté the onion until soft. Add the garlic and cook another two minutes.	
2	Add the diced potatoes and broth to the pot and bring to a boil. Reduce heat and simmer for about six minutes.	
3	Add the broccoli florets and cook for another 5-10 minutes, until both broccoli and potatoes are soft.	
4	Remove from the stove and use a heat-resistant immersion blender to puree the soup. This can be done in a blender, handling the hot soup with great care.	
5	Stir in the grated cheese and allow to melt. Return to low heat if necessary to melt the cheese. Salt and pepper to taste.	
6	Serve plain or garnished with more grated cheese, crumbled bacon or croutons.	

VEGGIE	**Vegetable Soup**^{V} **Serves 4-6**	**Soup**
INGREDIENTS		**SUBSTITUTE**
1	Onion, diced	
2 Tbsp	Butter	Extra Virgin Olive Oil or any light cooking oil
4-8 oz	Beef, diced (delete for vegetarian soup)	Any leftover beef steak or roast
32 oz	Beef broth	Vegetable broth
14.5 oz	Canned tomatoes, crushed	
¼ Head	Cabbage, finely sliced (about 2 C)	
2	Carrots, diced	
1 C	Corn, frozen or canned	
2	Potatoes, diced	
1 C	Green beans	Peas or lima beans
2 tsp	Italian seasoning	Basil or parsley
STEPS		
1	In a large stock pot, sauté the onion in the butter until it is soft.	
2	If using meat, uncooked meat may be browned with the onions. If using leftover meat (e.g. steak or roast), simply add it.	
3	Add all other ingredients and bring to a boil. Reduce heat and simmer for at least a half hour, longer if time allows. Salt and pepper to taste	

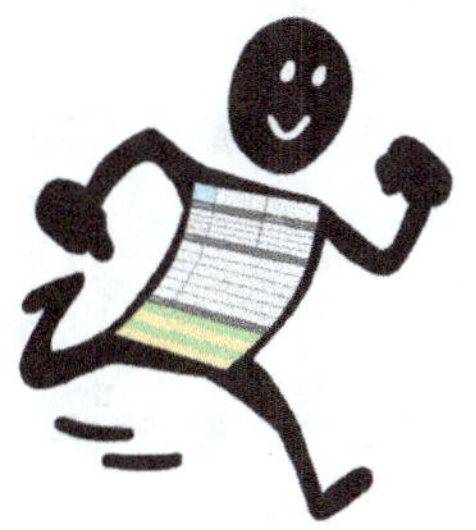

For more information and to download PDFs of Agile Recipes™ visit www.ReEngineeringtheKitchen.com.

Acknowledgments

This book was only possible with the help and support of many people but most of all my husband Harv. I need to thank him for his incredible patience and support – while writing this book and always. Cooking with Agile Recipes™ simply would not have come to fruition without his encouragement and making publication a priority. He was instrumental in every aspect from strategy to cooking to photography to project management.

Next, I need to acknowledge my illustrators. Simon Thompson created the cover design which creatively communicates the essence of the book at a glance. Guy Harvey brought the character "Agile" to life through his unique style of drawing.

I'd like to thank my publisher, White Bear Publishing, for faithfully bringing my vision to print in multiple formats. They did an exceptional job with the graphic design and layout. The innovative book layout was essential to presenting the new intuitive, one-page Agile Recipes™ format. Getting any cookbook, particularly Cooking with Agile Recipes™ with its extreme graphic requirements, to display effectively in an eBook format is nothing short of groundbreaking.

Lastly, I'd like to thank my family for their support and encouragement. They have provided the essential service of providing feedback and as recipe taste-testers for years. My daughters-in-law, Marisa and Eldis, have generously shared ideas, kitchen tips, and recipes. My grandsons, Erik and Reid, have helped in the test kitchen and, of course, taste testing. My amazing sons, Harvey and Brad, for always backing me in every endeavor. And of course, Smoky, my beloved English Cream Golden Retriever who happily provides moral support in the office and, especially, the kitchen.

INDEX

Keep up with the latest news and join the conversation on our website www.ReEngineeringtheKitchen.com

Download Agile Recipes™

Submit Agile Recipe™ Ideas

New Books in Progress

Read the Blog

About The Author

Alin (Alina) E. Steele

Alina writes nonfiction based on her life experiences and expertise including business, engineering, science, and food. She earned a BS in Chemical Engineering from Michigan State University and is a licensed Professional Engineer. She earned an MBA (Finance and Business Economics) from Wayne State University and a Certificate in Nutrition and Healthy Living from Cornell.

After a 30-year corporate career in the energy industry (and as a busy working mom), Alina now focuses on food and the related processes that we employ in our everyday lives. Agile Recipes™ were developed as part of Alina's first book Re-Engineering the Kitchen®, which focused on improving nutrition. The streamlined Agile Recipes™ with their one-page intuitive format were well received and led to the publication of Cooking with Agile Recipes™. You can find more information at www.reengineeringthekitchen.com.

Alina lives in Minnesota with her husband, Harv, and their amazing Golden Retriever, Smoky. She enjoys every adventure with her children and grandchildren and loves to visit friends in Florida or wherever they may be.

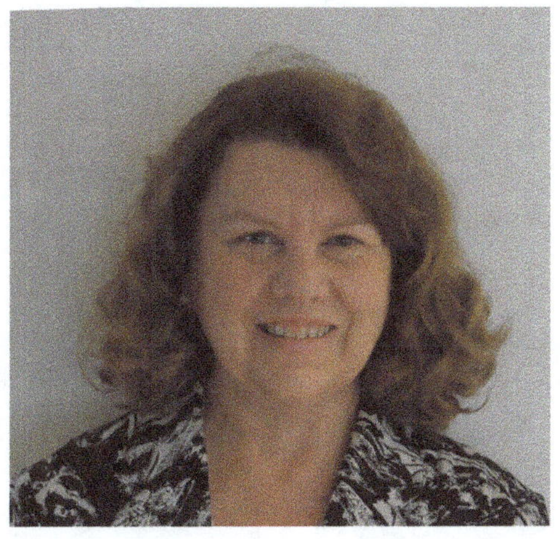

www.ingramcontent.com/pod-product-compliance
Lightning Source LLC
Chambersburg PA
CBHW080019130626
46556CB00016B/3227

* 9 7 9 8 9 8 9 3 4 7 5 5 1 *